DR. COLBERT'S
HEALTHY
GUT
ZONE

DON COLBERT, MD

SILOAM

Most Charisma House Book Group products are available at special quantity discounts for bulk purchase for sales promotions, premiums, fund-raising, and educational needs. For details, call us at (407) 333-0600 or visit our website at www.charismahouse.com.

DR. COLBERT'S HEALTHY GUT ZONE by Don Colbert, MD
Published by Siloam
Charisma Media/Charisma House Book Group
600 Rinehart Road, Lake Mary, Florida 32746

Illustrations by Abraham Mast

Visit the author's website at drcolbert.com, www.drcolbertbooks.com.

Library of Congress Cataloging-in-Publication Data:
An application to register this book for cataloging has been submitted to the Library of Congress.
International Standard Book Number: 978-1-62999-850-3
E-book ISBN: 978-1-62999-851-0

This book contains the opinions and ideas of its author. It is solely for informational and educational purposes and should not be regarded as a substitute for professional medical treatment. The nature of your body's health condition is complex and unique. Therefore, you should consult a health professional before you begin any new exercise, nutrition, or supplementation program or if you have questions about your health. Neither the author nor the publisher shall be liable or responsible for any loss or damage allegedly arising from any information or suggestion in this book.

21 22 23 24 25—9 8 7 6 5 4 3 2 1
Printed in the United States of America

CONTENTS

PREFACE

OVER THE PAST thirty-five-plus years, I can't tell you how many patients have come into my offices with a laundry list of symptoms:

- acid reflux
- arthritis
- bloating and gas
- brain fog
- chronic infections
- constant fatigue
- depression and anxiety
- joint aches
- loose stools
- migraines
- osteoporosis
- weight gain

Like most medical doctors, I was trained to quickly write a prescription so I could move on to the next patient. After all, that is the norm when seeing thirty to forty patients a day, and patients usually just want a pill to take so they can get on with their day.

The only problem was, nothing really changed. My patients might feel better for a little while, but often they came back with either a more severe case of the same symptoms or an entirely new set of challenges.

It was almost as if the prescriptions (antibiotics, stomach acid inhibitors, anti-inflammatory medications, etc.) were creating more problems than I was fixing. At least it seemed that way to me.

After years of this, my frustration grew. How could I be a doctor who "did no harm" if my patients were not getting better? The final push toward doing something different came when I was able to beat my own "incurable" and "permanent" case of psoriasis. The answers I found for myself, and thousands of patients since then, was not a prescription.

The primary answer had to do with the gut. Amazingly, the gut was the center of it all. The gut was the foundation of good health.

—DON COLBERT, MD

INTRODUCTION

THE GUT IS where most of the action is! It is the bedrock foundation of our health. Somehow the great physician Hippocrates (460–370 BC), the one responsible for the "do no harm" Hippocratic Oath that all doctors swear by, understood the importance of the gut. He is credited with saying, "All disease begins in the gut," and only recently are many of today's medical experts coming to the same conclusion.

But if you mention the importance and purpose of the gut, most people nod their heads knowingly. They have heard all about the gut's role in digestion, what to do if you have a stomachache, the importance of chewing your food properly, and how fiber can help with constipation.

That is like trekking through the vast Amazon jungle teeming with plants, trees, wildlife, insects, and unspeakable beauty only to say "It's humid" when asked to describe it. As it turns out, your gut is far more amazing that anyone expected, even trained medical doctors! Did you know the following facts?

- Your gut holds about one hundred trillion microbes (bacteria), and one drop of fluid from your colon contains more than a billion of these bacteria![1]

- If you want to lose weight, remember that your gut is responsible for telling your brain when you are full.[2] If that message is not delivered properly, you will still be hungry!

- If you battle anxiety or depression, it's helpful to know that 95 percent of your body's serotonin (the "happy chemical" that gives you a good mood) is in your gut![3] Is your gut doing its job?

- If you are trying to stay healthy, it's good to be aware that approximately 70–80 percent of your body's total immune cells are found in your gut![4] Is your gut healthy?

- If you struggle with brain fog or want to protect your brain from neurological diseases, know that there are one hundred million neurons in your gut that communicate with your brain![5] Is your gut inflamed and causing brain fog?

The gut plays more of a commanding role in disease prevention, weight loss, reversing sickness, and our overall health than we ever thought. Sadly, because we in the medical community did not know, many treatments have only hurt the gut more, and that has caused a lot of suffering, pain, disease, and even death.

I will outline a health plan in the following pages that will give your gut what it needs to benefit your body the most. Then the opposite of Hippocrates' concept that "all disease begins in the gut" can become a reality in your body: *all healing begins in the gut!*

PART I
GUT PROBLEMS

PART 1 EXPLAINS the purpose and power of the gut, along with the health problems that come when the gut wall is breached. What makes the gastrointestinal lining more permeable is entirely preventable. It is also imperative to your health that you take the necessary steps to get your gut healthy again.

CHAPTER ONE

THE HEALTHY GUT ZONE BEGINS

THE GUT ALWAYS seems to be the backstory, the proverbial "I didn't see that coming" if it were in a movie. For example, I can't tell you how many female patients I have treated over the years who complain about swelling, bloating, gas, and other bowel problems. As if that isn't enough, many of them are wearing shapewear! They eat and immediately swell up, sometimes followed by reflux (especially if shapewear is involved). They, of course, feel miserable, so they start taking antacids and then much stronger acid-suppressing drugs.

What may be happening is that when they eat excessive bread, fruit sugar, or starch after they have taken antibiotics, it usually ferments in their gut and produces hydrogen and methane gases. The swelling is often like a birthday balloon attached to a helium tank!

In the gut, specifically the small intestine, sometimes there is a war going on between beneficial, or "good," bacteria and harmful, or "bad," bacteria. The bad bacteria are usually winning, and the bloating and gas are simply symptoms of the conflict.

This discomfort is not the end of it. Doctors are quick to prescribe medication, typically with a ten-day to two-week prescription. Very quickly, the medicine becomes part of the regular daily routine, though the symptoms never go away.

The symptoms often get worse over time. Depending on the person, diarrhea or constipation is typically present, along with constant inflammation in the gut. It is the inflammation that causes untold damage, and it has a way of eventually spreading to the rest of the body.

One common diagnosis at this point is irritable bowel syndrome (IBS), though it is certainly not a news flash for those experiencing it. This condition can also be labeled as IBS-D (with diarrhea) or IBS-C (with constipation). The inflammation in the gut can cause either form of IBS.

When you stop the bloating and gas with medication, the result is usually something far worse. A damaged gut creates a host of other

3

symptoms, illnesses, and even diseases that make the initial symptoms pale in comparison.

However, if you treat the gut properly and get it healthy again, then usually the symptoms of swelling, bloating, gas, and other bowel problems eventually go away. A healthy gut will not only take care of your gut-related symptoms but also will often lessen and even eradicate a host of other ailments, even diseases!

As I said, the gut is far more powerful than we ever knew. It has the power to change your health and your life completely.

YOUR GUT

Your gut is your gastrointestinal tract (GI tract) and runs top to bottom, starting at your mouth, then extending through the esophagus, stomach, small intestine, and large intestine (colon) before ending at your rectum and anus—the last parts of your large intestine. The purpose of the gut has always been viewed as the digestion of food and absorption of nutrients, vitamins, minerals, simple sugars, fatty acids, and amino acids. What went in was either used or discarded. And there was nothing more to report.

Though not to the same degree as the French entertainer Michel Lotito, who ground up and ate bicycles, shopping carts, TV sets, beds, and even a small airplane,[1] it has been assumed for generations that our gut is pretty much indestructible. But that is not the case. Our gut is far less impervious or ironclad than we used to believe. This is so for two significant reasons:

1. **The gut is designed both to be permeable and to act as a barrier.** Absorbing nutrients, simple sugars, amino acids, fatty acids, vitamins, and minerals from the digested food into the bloodstream through the intestinal wall is part of the gut's job. It also acts as a barrier, preventing undigested foods, proteins, fats, and toxins from being absorbed.

2. **The gut can spring leaks.** An increasing number of proteins, foods, medicines, and bacteria have been found to, figuratively speaking, punch microscopic holes in the gut wall by damaging the tight junctions between the intestinal cells, allowing undigested food and toxins to leak through.

For us to simply live, our gut must provide us with nutrients from the foods we eat. But understandably, if excessive breaches (microscopic holes) occur in the gut, it becomes more permeable, meaning we develop a leaky gut (called increased intestinal permeability by many), and our health will naturally be compromised.

It makes sense, then, that your gut needs to be healthy for you to be healthy. After decades of treating patients, I have found this to be true. I have also found, generally speaking, that a healthy person has a healthy gut.

WHAT MAKES THE GUT SO SPECIAL?

Why is the gut so important, so special that it could play a role in our entire body's health? Or in "all disease" as Hippocrates argued?

That's a fair question. The answer is in what we don't see and until recently did not fully understand. More breakthroughs, Nobel prizes, and health options will come as a result of further research, but what we know so far makes a very compelling case for the gut being the center of health and wellness or sickness and disease.

IT'S A FACT

We all have two primary phyla of microbes in our gut: Firmicutes and Bacteroidetes. Excessive Firmicutes (F) make us fat; Bacteroidetes (B) help us stay lean. Your body needs the proper F/B ratio![2]

IT'S A FACT

"Microbial health is one of the factors that determines who survives potentially deadly viruses. The very young, whose microbiome is still developing, and the very old, who have fewer microbial species and less diversity, tend to be the most vulnerable."[3]

An excellent place to get a glimpse of the gut's importance is at the microscopic level. Here we can see what is happening on the inside.

Amazingly, your gut holds one hundred trillion microbes (bacteria), and each one has its own DNA.[4] These account for 90 percent of the total number of cells in your body![5] Yes, that means only 10 percent of your cells are human.

Most of these microbes are either harmless or beneficial for you. They provide an invaluable service, which includes breaking down indigestible food, supplying your gut with energy, making vitamins, breaking down toxins and medications, and training your immune system to defend itself.[6]

The trillions of microbes living in your gut comprise what is called a microbiome. If collected into a single jar, it would weigh up to five pounds and would consist primarily of these four phyla of bacteria: Actinobacteria, Proteobacteria, Firmicutes, and Bacteroidetes.[7] The latter two make up more than 90 percent of our gut microbes.[8]

We all have these microorganisms living in our gut (especially in the large intestine or colon) in differing amounts. Only recently have we found that this ratio or balance of microbes in the gut is a sign of good health or disease.

A healthy gut has a certain ratio, while an unhealthy gut has a different ratio. For example, thinner, healthier people usually have a gut ratio that is high in Bacteroidetes and low in Firmicutes, while it's the exact opposite with obese, unhealthy people.[9]

The question then becomes whether having the right ratio would improve our health, help us lose weight, and reduce or even remove many of the symptoms that we suffer from. Yes, that does happen. The gut is indeed special, far more important and powerful than we have ever known.

GUT PROBLEMS CAN BEGIN EARLY

When babies are born, they come down the birth canal and face-plant in their mothers' healthy vaginal and gut bacteria on the way out. This is good because that brief moment and small amount of fluid are enough for the microscopic bacteria to start to grow in the baby's tiny GI tract.

Then, as German doctor Giulia Enders points out, "Breastfeeding also promotes particular members of our gut flora—breast-milk-loving *Bifidobacteria*, for example. Colonizing the gut so early, these bacteria are instrumental in the development of later bodily functions, such as those of the immune system or the metabolic system. Children with insufficient

Bifidobacteria in their gut in their first year have an increased risk of obesity in later life."[10]

It is simply amazing how the normal and natural processes of birthing and breastfeeding are sufficient to jump-start the baby's microbiome with all its complexities, immune system, neurotransmitters, metabolism, health, and so much more. Yes, it truly is!

You may be wondering about babies born via C-section who miss the brief bacterial bath with their mother. That is a very real concern. Researchers have found some startling results for babies born via C-section. Here are two quick examples: The average asthma rate in the US for children is 8.4 percent, but with C-section births, the rate is 9.5 percent. Average obesity rates for children are around 16 percent but over 19 percent with C-section births.[11]

These trends continue. C-section babies also have an increased risk of

- attention deficit hyperactivity disorder (ADHD),[12]
- allergies,[13]
- autism,[14]
- celiac disease,[15] and
- type 1 diabetes.[16]

Unfortunately, there is an increasing global trend toward C-section births. Well over 50 percent of births are done via C-section in several countries, including Dominican Republic, Brazil, Egypt, Turkey, and Cyprus. C-sections account for greater than 40 percent of births in nations such as Chile, Iran, Mexico, and Romania and more than 30 percent in numerous European countries and the United States.[17]

IT'S A FACT

You need your gut bacteria because of all these things they do for you:

» *Breaking down food so your body can absorb it*[18]

» *Making chemicals to curb inflammation*[19]

» *Strengthening your gut wall to protect you from harmful bacteria*[20]

» *Identifying which bacteria are bad and alerting the immune system*[21]

» *Helping immune cells develop*[22]

» *Helping to balance hormones*[23]

Does it make a difference if a baby is born naturally or via C-section? Does the initial ingesting of good bacteria benefit the baby all that much? In the eye-opening book *Gut Crisis*, authors R. Keith and Samantha Wallace clearly state, "If our immune system is deprived of this early education, we are far more likely to develop a wide range of diseases."[24]

Nobody signs up for a "wide range of diseases," but as a medical doctor, I wonder why anyone would risk it. Of course, there are times when a C-section birth is needed for the mother's or baby's well-being, but afterward, things can be done to strengthen and grow the baby's microbiome, with breastfeeding being the optimum choice.

Going into adulthood, a lot of us started at a disadvantage. Through no fault of our own, our gut balance—the ratio of good to bad bacteria—was off. And our bodies paid a price for it that we are only now understanding.

From our first breath, the gut plays a vital role in every single aspect of our lives. Be it our brains, metabolism, immunity, skin, or feelings, it's all affected by the gut. And if that's not enough, even our DNA can be altered by the state of our gut![25]

Thankfully our overall health is not based solely on how we were born. It does play a part, but it is not the end of the story. How we started out matters a great deal, but how we eat and live from today forward is much more important.

The point is, your gut plays a primary role in your current and future health. Treat it well, make it healthy, and you will reap the many benefits.

CHAPTER TWO

CAN THE GUT HAVE PROBLEMS?

WHEN I STARTED in medicine as a solo practitioner, trying to meet the needs of thirty to forty patients each day was intense. There was no time to be sick. But I was under pressure to grow the business, meet payroll, pay the mortgage, cover car payments, keep the whole process moving, and more.

IT'S A FACT

Your gut wall uses about 40 percent of your total body energy expenditure, whereas the brain uses only 20 percent. The gut wall is a busy place and vitally important to your health.[1]

Have you ever been too busy to get sick? As you know, that usually doesn't end well. For me, as I ran myself ragged, my immune system would get more and more run down. I would invariably get sick with a sinus infection or bronchitis. This would happen every three to four months.

As soon as I developed symptoms, I would take an antibiotic. After completing the regimen of antibiotics for seven to ten days, I would feel great. Then several months later, I would get sick again and repeat the antibiotic process.

This went on for years. Eventually, I developed IBS because I had unintentionally killed off many of the good bacteria in my gut with the antibiotics. But I didn't know it at the time.

Diarrhea four or five times a day was my new normal. Then it got worse a few years later. I developed psoriasis all over my arms, legs, and hands. The itchy rash kept me from sleeping. Simply put, my body was a mess!

It was then that I set to work to find out what was wrong with my body. I found the foods that triggered inflammation in my body. I changed my diet. The psoriasis eventually cleared up, but it took a few more years for me to figure out how to beat the IBS.

The journey was a long one, but it was a trip I never really had to take! I didn't know it at the time, but the "new normal" of diarrhea from IBS was not a normal life at all! Nor was the getting sick every few months, antibiotic cycle, inflammation, or psoriasis.

Eventually, I figured it out: if I have a healthy gut, then I will be healthy as well.

Your Gut Affects It All

How is it that the gut plays such a massive role in our overall health? It might seem a little outrageous to some people that the GI tract, which is about thirty feet long and runs from mouth to anus, is all that important to every part of our lives. That is understandable. At one level, it does seem illogical that the mouth, esophagus, stomach, small intestine, and large intestine can affect the brain, immune system, heart, body weight, and overall health.

But imagine you have run a hot bath and are preparing for a relaxing soak after a long, hard day. A live electrical wire runs right through the water, but you have been assured that the wire has no holes. Would you get in the tub? Or suppose you find out that the local water purification plant in your area has large metal pipes of raw sewage running directly through the holding tank of fresh water. They guarantee the aged, rusty pipes do not leak. How thirsty are you now?

Just like a wire or a pipe, your gut can develop holes or spring leaks, and that is only one of the problems. Another issue is the fact that what we put into our mouths in the form of foods, beverages, and medications can kill off so much of the good bacteria in the gut that it takes years to regrow.

The proven and potential effects cannot be ignored because they come in the form of symptoms, ailments, sicknesses, and diseases. All of this comes through the doctor's door at one time or another. The following list is a snapshot of what I have seen on a daily basis for many years. All these have one thing in common: a healthy gut can bring relief, improve, reduce, and sometimes heal every one of them!

Brain

- ADHD
- Alzheimer's disease
- autism
- brain fog
- dementia
- memory problems
- Parkinson's disease
- Tourette's syndrome

Lung, heart, and mouth

- asthma
- atherosclerosis
- gum disease
- halitosis
- heart disease
- high blood pressure

Body

- allergies
- arthritis
- chronic fatigue
- chronic yeast problems
- diabetes
- extreme menstrual and menopausal symptoms
- fibromyalgia
- food sensitivities
- joint and muscle inflammation
- obesity
- slow metabolism

Autoimmune

- Graves' disease
- Hashimoto's thyroiditis
- lupus
- multiple sclerosis
- rheumatoid arthritis
- vitiligo

Skin

- acne
- dermatitis
- eczema
- lichen planus
- psoriasis

Mood and sleep

- anxiety
- depression
- insomnia
- mood swings

Gut

- acid reflux
- chronic constipation or diarrhea
- Crohn's disease
- gas and bloating
- inflammatory bowel disease
- small intestinal bacterial overgrowth (SIBO)
- small intestinal fungal overgrowth (SIFO)
- ulcerative colitis
- ulcers

What is pretty incredible—even amazing—is watching patients with one or more items on this list improve by getting their guts healthy again. I have seen patients' symptoms eradicated, medications discontinued, and diseases cured.

Noted neurologist Dr. David Perlmutter went so far as to say that "up to 90 percent of all known human illness can be traced back to an unhealthy gut. And we can say for sure that just as disease begins in the gut, so too does health and vitality."[2] It only makes sense. If you can restore the gut to a healthy condition, then the body will usually match that state of good health.

That's what happens in the gut when the good bacteria outnumber the bad. More and more medical experts are acknowledging that the condition of our gut's microbiome speaks volumes about our current and future health.

A healthy gut is what you want! Usually, however, the opposite is the case. Our symptoms often match the unhealthy state of our gut.

There is no single comprehensive test to gauge the health level of your gut and its microbiome. However, the previous list of symptoms, ailments, sicknesses, and diseases is a telltale sign of your gut health. If you suffer from anything on that list, then your gut health probably needs improving.

Because your gut's microbiome has grown since you were born, even since you were conceived, it reflects everything that has happened to you. Take a minute to complete this chart, taken from Dr. Perlmutter's book *Brain Maker:*[3]

	Yes	No
Did your mother take antibiotics while she was pregnant with you?		
Were you born by C-section?		
Were you breastfed for less than one month?		
Did you suffer from frequent ear or throat infections as a child?		
Did you require ear tubes as a child?		
Did you have your tonsils removed?		
Do you take antibiotics at least once every two to three years?		

	Yes	No
Do you take acid-blocking drugs (for digestion or reflux)?		
Are you gluten-sensitive?		
Do you have food allergies?		
Are you extra sensitive to chemicals often found in everyday products and goods?		
Have you been diagnosed with an autoimmune disease?		
Do you suffer from irritable bowel syndrome?		
Do you have diarrhea or loose bowel movements at least once a month?		
Do you suffer from depression?		

You go to the doctor because you are suffering from something. That is only natural. I would say that virtually every patient who goes to a doctor, regardless of the person's sickness or ailment, usually has a problem in his or her gut. I can't tell you how many patients found relief when we got their guts healthy again.

I would also go so far as to say this: if everyone had a healthy gut, most doctors would instantly be out of business. Only having ten patients out of a thousand would change things considerably! But that is certainly not happening anytime soon. The rates for sickness and disease, especially for the more than eighty autoimmune disorders and the twenty-five or more obesity-linked health conditions out there today,[4] have been rising for decades.

The answers are in the gut.

THE THREE DOMINOES OF GUT PROBLEMS

It is important to understand the domino effect of the gut. The weakening process does not just happen suddenly. It happens over time, one domino at a time.

Domino 1: Early gut problems

First, as already mentioned, the gut may initially be weakened by how we were birthed, what we were fed, and whether we were medicated. We

Rhea,
our library
dog says ...

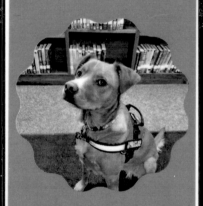

... just keep
reading

412 Budd St.
Carthage, NY
13619

315-493-2620
carlib@ncls.org

Thank you
for playing
Virtual Bingo!

Follow us on Facebook to see
upcoming events
Facebook.com/CarthageFreeLibrary

will discuss medications in greater detail in future chapters, but these three factors are the beginning.

Domino 2: Daily choices

Second, we make daily choices about what we eat, how we live, what medications we take, what we drink, and much more. All this adds up to create issues in the gut, and the gut usually becomes more permeable or starts to leak. We will also discuss this in greater detail in coming chapters.

Domino 3: Foods we eat

Third, what we eat after the gut has started to leak creates a world of suffering, pain, discomfort, and disease. Those are all the symptoms that come into doctors' offices every day. This will be explained soon in greater detail.

The point is, when we have symptoms that match the earlier list of ailments and diseases, they are almost always the combined result of all the health choices we made up to that point. Granted, some choices may have been out of our control and some may even be genetic, but they still apply. The dominoes have fallen.

Thankfully, you can tip the dominoes back up again.

CHAPTER THREE

HOW THE GUT STARTS TO LEAK

THE SYMPTOMS ARE not the root cause. Every doctor knows that, but many times the root cause is hard to find. When Robert came into my office complaining about memory-related issues and saying his dad had dementia, I knew there had to be more to the conversation than just genetics.

> ## IT'S A FACT
>
> *Did you know: The bacteria in your gut "help determine which diseases are expressed, turning various human genes on and off in response to the body's internal milieu, which can influence whether or not a disease that you're genetically predisposed to actually develops."*[1]

Most doctors agree with the gene-environment-trigger approach, which argues that most sickness and disease are brought about in this way:

1. We have *genes* that predispose us to specific ailments.

2. We form an *environment* around us by what we eat, how we live, how much we exercise or how active we are, what choices we make, etc.

3. A *trigger* causes the symptoms to erupt, leading to the impending sickness or disease.

In other words, your genetics may "load the gun," but it's usually your environment (stress, food choices, lifestyle) that pulls the trigger and sets off the disease. But doctors usually don't agree on what one's environment causes, what the triggers might be, or what symptoms mean. Also, doctors probably don't know the genetic markers for each of their patients. This is why you can expect to hear conflicting reasons for the very same symptoms!

Robert's first doctor visit led to a pretty grim prognosis: better prepare for dementia. Though Robert did have a family member with dementia, this did not necessarily mean he had dementia, much less the actual genes commonly associated with it.

We started by looking at a list of potential triggers and environmental factors, trying to work our way backward. When you remove the trigger or triggers and remedy the environment, the symptoms will usually go away. I have seen many diagnosed diseases cured completely after taking these steps.

That was what happened to Robert. After changing his diet (discussed in full in the coming chapters), which included adding such things as prebiotics, probiotics, fiber, healthy fats, and low-carb foods, along with going gluten-free, his early dementia symptoms cleared up.

It has been several years, and Robert is doing fine.

THE SYMPTOMS ARE NOT THE PROBLEM

Nobody puts an adhesive bandage on a thorn. Naturally, you pull out the thorn first. But honestly speaking, this illogical treatment happens all the time—and in the name of "do no harm," no less.

Consider the following list from Dr. Steven R. Gundry.[2] I promise you that when patients visit their doctors with these symptoms, they almost always receive medicine to treat the symptom, but the root problem goes untreated.

- aching joints
- acid reflux or heartburn
- acne
- age spots
- allergies
- alopecia
- anemia
- arthritis

- asthma
- autoimmune diseases (thyroid disease, rheumatoid arthritis, type 1 diabetes, multiple sclerosis, Crohn's, colitis, lupus)
- bone loss (osteopenia and osteoporosis)
- brain fog
- cancer
- canker sores
- chronic fatigue syndrome
- chronic pain syndrome
- colon polyps
- cramps, tingling, numbness
- decline in dental health
- dementia
- depression
- diabetes, prediabetes, insulin resistance
- dizziness
- ear ringing
- exhaustion
- fibromyalgia
- gastroesophageal reflux disease (GERD)
- gastrointestinal problems (bloating, pain, gas, constipation, diarrhea)
- headaches
- heart disease
- hypertension
- IBS
- infertility
- irregular menstrual cycle
- irritability
- low testosterone
- low white blood cell count

- lymphomas
- malabsorption like low iron
- male-pattern baldness
- memory loss
- migraine headaches
- Parkinson's disease
- peripheral neuropathy
- skin rashes
- skin tags
- vitiligo
- weight gain
- weight loss

Dr. Gundry has found that when you fix the gut, all these symptoms usually clear up! He argues that the root cause of most diseases is in the gut, and I have also found that to be the case.

For decades, both doctors and patients have been so focused on the symptoms that we've missed the underlying problems. And as you know, treating symptoms seldom cures anything.

Pull the thorn out! When you treat the root cause, the symptoms will usually go away.

IT'S A FACT

Weight gain is one of the most common side effects of a leaky gut.

START WITH YOUR SYMPTOMS

Symptoms are what people notice first and what makes them aware that something is out of order inside their bodies. Take a moment and look carefully at Dr. Gundry's list of symptoms and disorders above. Do you have any of those symptoms or diseases? If you have had one or more, did you go to a doctor? What prescription were you given? And have your symptoms gone away? Have new symptoms developed since you started taking the prescribed medication? Answering these questions will give you greater clarity about your health.

Looking at averages, 69 percent of American and Canadian adults from ages forty to seventy-nine take one or more prescriptions, and 22 percent take five or more prescribed medications. The most common prescriptions include antidepressants, cholesterol-reducing drugs, and hypertension or heart-related medicines.[3]

Think about that for just a second! I have found from experience that people take most medications over an extended period because the symptoms usually don't go away. Patients request new prescriptions, doctors keep writing them out, and the cycle continues.

But do you know what is causing your symptoms? That is perhaps *the* most important question to have answered. Hopefully, we will be able to find that answer in the following pages and also spell out a game plan to remove those symptoms. Almost every disease—from depression to anxiety, obesity, autoimmune disease, or heart disease—and the related symptoms that go with so many ailments are associated with the health of your gut.

Not only have we as a society treated the symptoms, but we have also missed the root cause by a mile. And if that is not enough, we have been causing the problem or making it worse by the very foods we eat, the medications we take, and the lifestyle we choose to live.

As a direct result of decades of this "treat the symptom, not the root" approach to life and medicine, we are experiencing a dramatic increase in preventable diseases, billions of dollars wasted, and lives spent coping with illness instead of thriving.

IT'S A FACT

"Inflammation is the root cause of most chronic diseases, including cardiovascular disease, arthritis, Alzheimer's disease, Parkinson's disease, most cancers, autoimmune disease (such as rheumatoid arthritis, lupus, MS, colitis, Crohn's disease), and more."[4]

Yes, the symptoms are real, but they are usually a sign that something is wrong in the gut. The underlying problem is usually this: you have a leaky gut, which is an increase in intestinal permeability. This is the foundational cause of countless sicknesses, diseases (including autoimmune diseases), ailments, inflammation, pains, weight gain, and discomfort. You name it, and a leaky gut is most likely the cause. Consider this from Dr. Gundry:

> Although…I originally thought that leaky gut was an isolated condition affecting a few unfortunate individuals, now I am convinced that leaky gut underlies all our disease issues, just as Hippocrates posited.[5]

WHAT EXACTLY IS A LEAKY GUT?

Part of the gut's primary job is to break down the nutrients from what you eat into simple sugars, amino acids, fatty acids, vitamins, and minerals and absorb them into your body so you get the benefits of what you have eaten. The actual absorption process happens in two different ways: *through* the cells (transcellular) or *between* the cells (paracellular) of your gut wall.[6]

A leaky gut can also be called increased gut permeability or increased intestinal permeability. But whatever it's called, these gut issues have to do with problems that occur between the cells. When the microscopic tight junctions between these cells of the gut wall are damaged and pried open, the result is tiny holes that let bacteria, proteins, partially digested food, chemicals, yeast, toxins, and more directly into your bloodstream![7]

Inflammation is the inevitable result of these many small leaks. And unfortunately for your body, inflammation is the root cause of most chronic diseases and virtually every symptom on the list you read a few pages ago!

That's right. The entire list, from the symptoms to the full-blown diseases, is the result of a leaky gut. Fix the gut, and it will usually go away? Apparently so! Everything on that list from Dr. Gundry also describes patients he has successfully treated. When they fixed the gut, their problems went away.[8]

Part of the challenge in the gut is that the purpose of the gut wall is to let nutrients, vitamins, simple sugars, and enzymes pass through and into the body. That's how the body is made to work. If it were an impermeable pipe, you would starve to death even while having a full stomach!

IT'S A FACT

These are your four defenses against viruses and bacteria:

1. mucus in your nose and saliva in your mouth

2. stomach acid

3. beneficial bacteria in your mouth and gut

4. the layer of mucus produced in your intestines[9]

Another challenge is that the lining of your small intestine is only one cell thick and has the surface area of a small studio apartment (up to 430 square feet)![10] This entire area is simultaneously under attack by the food we eat, the medications we take, and the lifestyle we choose.

The result is that the tight junctions between the cells of the gut wall are pried open just enough to let the wrong things through. Imagine taking your coffee filter and poking holes in it with a fork. Naturally, your next cup of coffee would be full of coffee grounds.

What's happening to your gut wall is similar. When many microscopic holes appear, inflammation begins, food sensitivities occur, health problems arise, and more holes appear, etc. Things get exponentially worse over time.

HOW TO FIX A LEAKY GUT

I have had many patients who displayed many of the same symptoms listed earlier in this chapter. Every symptom is usually a telltale sign of a leaky gut. When we healed their leaky guts, they usually found the relief, fix, or cure they needed.

In its briefest form (to be explained in complete detail in the following chapters), there are two basic steps to fixing a leaky gut:

1. **Step 1: Get rid of the bad.** Remove offending foods, bad or excessive bacteria and yeast, parasites, medications, toxins, and more. Learn to cope with stress.

2. **Step 2: Eat more of the good.** Recharge the gut with good bacteria in the form of probiotics and sometimes prebiotics, and regularly eat foods that support the gut.

That's it in a nutshell. When you remove the things that trigger a leaky gut and then recharge the gut with healthy foods, you will be amazed how your gut can heal. I have seen some pretty severe health situations start to turn around in as little as two weeks. More often, it takes four to six weeks for an undeniable change to take place, and within three months, the symptoms are usually gone or greatly reduced.

IT'S A FACT

Your gut is smart. It memorizes invader molecules so that if they return, the body can respond more quickly.[11]

All that to say, keeping your gut healthy is probably the best thing you can do for your overall and long-term health.

All this effort for a microscopic hole in the gut? No, a leaky gut is not about a single tiny hole in the gut wall or even a few holes. Multiple millions of cells join together to form the gut lining.[12] So a leaky gut could have thousands or even millions of microscopic holes or more, depending on the severity of the leaky gut, each hole allowing molecules into your body that cause inflammation and sickness. This is not about one hole!

Big holes in the gut from ulcers are well researched, painful, and potentially deadly, but it wasn't until recently that we discovered how many smaller holes a gut can have. Much of the inflammation and discomfort, sickness and disease people live with now makes sense. We know why it's happening, and we know how to fix it. And when we fix a leaky gut, health usually returns to the body!

CHAPTER FOUR

SEVEN CAUSES OF A LEAKY GUT

Osteoporosis is like a slow-motion slide toward debilitation and eventual hospitalization. Several years ago, an older woman came into my offices. She was suffering from osteoporosis and osteoarthritis. She was in chronic pain. I was worried about bone loss and eventually breaking bones that would limit her freedom. She lived at home alone and enjoyed her independence.

IT'S A FACT

What you eat and how you treat your body have a direct cause-and-effect relationship on your health, immune system, mood, neurological function, and more. Treat your good bacteria well, and they will take good care of you.[1]

As we talked, she explained how she had been taking antacids for years. Both she and her husband, who passed away a few years earlier, regularly took antacid pills and then took a proton pump inhibitor—the little purple pills known as Prilosec.

"It's been at least twenty years," she said. "We first thought it was spicy foods, but then it was most foods after dinner that upset our stomachs, so we made it a practice to always take antacids and eventually Prilosec."

She had succeeded in eliminating stomach acid, but in so doing, she had also limited her gut's ability to absorb calcium, magnesium, and other nutrients from the foods she ate and supplements she took. Her osteoporosis was a direct result of twenty years of trying to suppress stomach acid.

"You need your stomach acid," I explained, "but certainly not heartburn and reflux."

So she started this regimen to increase her good gut bacteria:

- eating foods and taking supplements that repaired her gut
- supplementing the minerals and nutrients that her body (especially her bones and joints) needed, including collagen, vitamin D_3, vitamin K_2, calcium, magnesium, etc.
- taking natural anti-inflammatory supplements (curcumin and Boswellia)
- taking several other healthy steps to improve her quality of life, including specific exercises

Within a month, her joint inflammation had noticeably decreased, and eventually, she was able to wean herself off her antacid medications. The more she ate the right gut-friendly foods, the better she felt. At her yearly checkup, her bone density was improving rather than decreasing as it had been for many years.

She kept at it, and after a couple of years, she no longer has osteoporosis and is still doing great and living independently. She is now busier than ever before, doing more activities than she would have thought possible when we first met. Fixing her gut was the answer she had been looking for.

THE SEVEN CAUSES OF A LEAKY GUT

Do you know why your gut leaks? What is the underlying reason that you might suffer from one or many of the symptoms on the previous pages? The answer is in your gut.

IT'S A FACT

Increasing certain good bacteria in the gut can help you lose weight.[2]

Research has shown what doctors see every day in their offices—the most common causes of a leaky gut. The causes that I see are as follows, from most common to least:

1. antibiotics
2. NSAIDs

3. acid-blocking meds

4. GMO foods

5. chlorine in drinking water

6. pesticides

7. intestinal infections

These usually cause the gut wall to begin to leak. Once that happens, many of the typical foods we eat may make the situation worse. Consuming foods that you are unknowingly sensitive to causes even more inflammation in the gut. As a direct result, the bad bacteria in the gut often increase exponentially, and that reduces the good bacteria. In other words, we can say that many times leaky gut is due to chronic inflammation. If the root cause is not addressed, it is unlikely that your medical conditions can improve.

Because of the leaky gut, inflammation is typically rampant. Your body reacts to foods that you are not allergic to because the leaky gut leads to increased food sensitivities that lead to inflammation that eventually lead to sickness and disease. It's those dominoes again. (We will discuss ten common enemies of the gut, including gluten, in chapter 6.)

And then, if you don't heal the gut, all the inflammation and gut-related issues begin to affect your brain negatively! If that isn't motivating enough, did you know that a leaky gut is "a precondition for developing an autoimmune disease since it's the increase in intestinal permeability—the opening of the door from our gut into our body—that allows toxins to enter and then trigger an immune response"?[3]

For decades we have medicated rather than fixed the real issues. It has been the normal procedure in doctors' offices across the country and around the world, but we are finding that every major disease is usually connected back to the gut. And when the gut wall is compromised, the entire body is at risk.

When someone is sick, obese, or diagnosed with a disease, his or her gut is usually not healthy. Only rarely will you find a healthy gut in an unhealthy person. Instead, the gut is a reflection of what's going on in the rest of the body.

First things first: before we can talk about health, losing weight, or giving the body the food it needs, we must first stop the gut from leaking or improve intestinal permeability. Only after the gut stops leaking will the body usually be able to heal itself.

What does a leaky gut look like? First, you must understand what a healthy gut looks like and why.

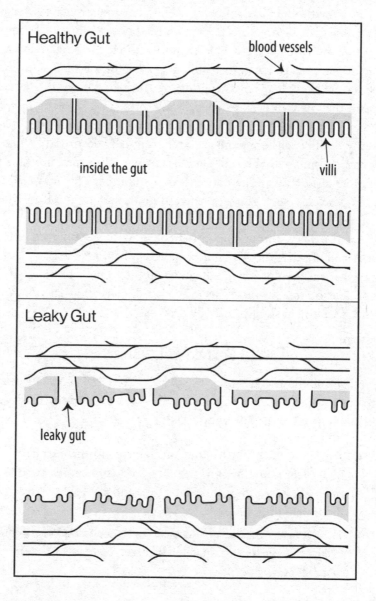

As the illustration of a healthy gut shows, the gut wall is made of cells that have little villi (tiny, fingerlike projections) on one side (the side that touches the food you eat), and on the other side, it has blood vessels that feed directly into your bloodstream. The villi play a vital role in the absorption of amino acids, fatty acids, nutrients, and sugars from what you eat. Everything is broken down to minute simple sugars, fatty acids, and amino acids before absorption into the body is allowed. Whole proteins from food are naturally blocked until sufficiently broken down.

But when damage happens in the gut, some of the little villi are flattened or broken off. The disruption of the villi allows the junctions between the gut wall cells to open; whole proteins and other molecules can then pass through, causing inflammation, sickness, and then disease.

Many healthy cells are damaged and eventually destroyed. When this happens, the microvilli are not able to do their job, which prevents your body from absorbing all the nutrients that you need. This may lead to all sorts of problems, such as a weakened immune system, inflammation, or nutritional deficiencies.

We will discuss throughout this book how to return your gut to a healthy condition again. The following seven causes of a leaky gut may reveal what has been secretly damaging your gut. I hope not only that you will be able to protect yourself from further damage but that you can also get the relief and healing your body deserves.

CAUSE 1 OF LEAKY GUT: ANTIBIOTICS

The most common cause of a leaky gut that I see is the overuse of antibiotics—whether from the prescriptions we take or the food we eat. Did you know all of the following facts?

- The US is one of the leading antibiotic consumers among high-income countries.[4] In 2016, US doctors wrote over 270 million prescriptions for antibiotics, and at least 30 percent of these were unnecessary.[5]
- The average American child receives ten courses of antibiotics by age ten and approximately seventeen courses by the time he or she turns twenty.[6]

- For decades, antibiotics have been used to fatten farm animals. When we eat those antibiotic-fed animals, the same fattening process may be happening to us.[7]

Remember that the gut can start at a disadvantage due to C-section births and lack of breastfeeding. With C-section births, many mothers are given antibiotics to ward off infections, but this practice risks the babies' exposure to the antibiotics. And that is not good.[8] Consider this:

- The use of antibiotics at a young age can predispose a child to such conditions as allergies, asthma, autoimmune diseases, mental health disorders, and obesity.[9]
- Every dose of antibiotics increases a child's risk of developing asthma, Crohn's disease, diabetes, or obesity.[10]

What are the antibiotics doing to your body? Antibiotics, designed to kill off bad bacteria or pathogens that are causing sickness or infection, do so in three different ways: "by peppering the bacteria with holes, by poisoning the bacteria, or by rendering the bacteria unable to reproduce."[11]

IT'S A FACT

The livestock and poultry industry uses 80 percent of the antibiotics sold in the US.[12]

The problem is that with each dose, the good bacteria are put through the same regimen, and they die along with the bad. A single course of antibiotics is enough to mess up your good gut bacteria for an entire year![13]

I seldom prescribe antibiotics, and I always recommend that you explore other options, get a second opinion, or take a natural antibiotic. However, there are times when your body does need antibiotics to fight off sickness.

IT'S A FACT

If your gut bacteria are out of balance, you usually have dysbiosis, which means you have inadequate beneficial bacteria present in your gut and excessive bad bacteria.

In some situations, if they are indeed required, I suggest getting antibiotics that are specific and not broad-spectrum. The broad-spectrum antibiotics created in the 1960s and 1970s effectively kill many strains of bacteria and have saved many lives, but they still do incredible damage to your gut wall.[14] My recommendation is that you avoid broad-spectrum antibiotics unless you are dangerously sick. This type of antibiotic can hurt the gut for years, and sometimes the damage is permanent.

The secondary problem is that we overuse antibiotics, viewing them as supposed miracle cures to treat anything and everything that afflicts us. This overzealous antibiotic use puts our gut health—and thus our overall health—at risk.

A good example of this is the when-in-doubt-take-an-antibiotic approach to the common cold. When someone has a cold, antibiotics are often prescribed. But did you know that viruses—*not* bacteria—cause all colds, which means the antibiotic does no good at all? Antibiotics have no effect on a virus. In fact, they will have a significant negative impact on the gut by killing off a large number of good bacteria. Clearly not a good move! Maybe the bacteria will grow back, and maybe they won't. But whenever good bacteria are killed off, your body takes a hit for a period of time.

Think of it this way: your good bacteria perform countless tasks all day long that help you, your immune system, your gut, and your health, which all depend on these bacteria. If you suddenly remove a significant portion of your good bacteria, that means your immune system and health will invariably be affected.

IT'S A FACT

Diarrhea is a common reaction to antibiotics.

Typically, weight gain is gradual, brain fog increases, symptoms begin to pile up, and everything slowly gets worse. Until the good bacteria are reintroduced or nursed back to health, it's going to be a losing battle.

IT'S A FACT

An estimated 30 percent of all antibiotic prescriptions in the US are for illnesses that do not require an antibiotic.[15]

That's why leaky gut is credited as being the root cause of most diseases. And it's why gastroenterologist Dr. Robynne Chutkan recommends, "Avoidance of antibiotics is absolutely the number one strategy for keeping your microbiome healthy."[16] I agree with her.

Alternatives/options/choices

Thankfully, there are other options. For example, if a woman has symptoms of a urinary tract infection (UTI), I culture the urine and immediately start her on a natural supplement called D-mannose (made from cranberry) of two to four tablets (500 mg each) twice a day. It does no harm. Usually the culture shows there is no infection, which means she can stop taking D-mannose.

Another herb called cat's-claw, one capsule (500 mg) three times a day, can be used for viral upper respiratory infections, colds, and ear infections. And it's readily available in most health-food stores.

If an infection turns out to be bacterial, I may use a narrow-spectrum antibiotic for seven days to kill the specific bacteria causing the infection. This does the least harm to the gut and the good bacteria. Or patients can go to the health-food store and purchase Silver Biotics (not colloidal silver), which kills bacteria, viruses, fungus, and yeast.

Rather than simply taking antibiotics out of habit, work with a doctor who will address your symptoms from as natural an approach as possible. Try to avoid antibiotics if you can, and utilize the countless natural supplements and herbs that are readily available these days for infections. Patients need to think about these two questions:

1. Before you take antibiotics, are you sure the sickness is bacterial?

2. Will the damage to your gut exceed the benefits of the antibiotic?

The more I treat patients who have overused antibiotics during their lifetimes, the more I highly recommend that they consider other options rather than requesting an antibiotic prescription. Almost always, the gut damage from antibiotics is much worse than the sickness was in the first place.

I can't tell them what to do; they get to decide. Likewise, it's your health, so you get to choose.

Cause 2 of Leaky Gut: NSAIDs

The second biggest cause of a leaky gut is something that will probably surprise most people. Have you taken any of these?

- aspirin
- celecoxib (Celebrex)
- ibuprofen (Motrin, Advil)
- meloxicam (Mobic)
- naproxen (Aleve, Naprosyn)
- another nonsteroidal anti-inflammatory drug (NSAID)

Though they may bring temporary relief to pain, in return, they usually cause even greater damage than the pain relief was worth by damaging the gut wall and increasing gut permeability.[17]

IT'S A FACT

A leaky gut often causes your body to react to foods that you are not even sensitive or allergic to.

These are nonsteroidal anti-inflammatory drugs or NSAIDs. Created in the 1970s as another option for aspirin, it turns out that, even in low doses, they damage your gut.[18] According to experts, NSAIDs do the following to your gut wall:

- NSAIDs "blow gaping holes in the mucus-lined intestinal barrier."[19]
- NSAIDs block prostaglandins, which can cause complications such as ulcers, "bleeding, perforation, stricture,...iron deficiency anemia and protein loss."[20]
- NSAIDs "can cause ulceration and increase the intestinal permeability of the lining of the gut, which allows bacteria to translocate through and damage the mucosa—a major contributor to the phenomenon of a leaky gut."[21]

In other words, they hurt the mucus layer of your gut by dissolving microscopic holes through your gut wall. These are mini versions of ulcers. In the same way that aspirin taken on an empty stomach can create craters and holes in the gut wall, so, too, do NSAIDs.

As a result of the damage done to the gut wall, inflammation flares up. That is the natural result, and it leads directly to a leaky gut!

Unfortunately, you may eventually need to take more NSAIDs to treat the same symptoms, and that only makes things worse. In addition, you usually have to contend with more gut damage.

Alternatives/options/choices

As you may have guessed, NSAIDs are always one of the top-selling pharmaceutical prescriptions. Yet two great alternatives to NSAIDs are a combination of curcumin and Boswellia (both readily available in most health-food stores). They help reduce inflammation as well as or better than other anti-inflammatory medications without damaging the gut. I usually recommend taking one to two 500 mg capsules of curcumin twice a day with one to two 100 mg capsules of Boswellia AKBA (or 5-LOXIN) twice a day.

CAUSE 3 OF LEAKY GUT: ACID BLOCKERS

Like NSAIDs, the next prominent cause of a leaky gut is taking a medication that fixes one problem while creating another.

> ### IT'S A FACT
>
> *"Antacids cause leaky gut by suppressing digestion of your food, making it more likely that your immune system will be triggered by the food you eat."*[22]

> ### IT'S A FACT
>
> *By suppressing stomach acid, you are giving the bad bacteria in your gut free rein to cause a lot of damage.*

Acid-blocking drugs are a significant player in causing leaky gut. Whether prescribed or purchased without a prescription, acid blockers treat heartburn, acid reflux, GERD, and other acid-related symptoms, such as ulcer disease, gastritis, and more. The immediate goal is to reduce stomach acid. The following acid blockers are commonly used:

- Dexilant
- Nexium
- Prevacid
- Prilosec
- Protonix
- Zegerid

However, the big problem here is the simple fact that your body needs stomach acid to function properly. Digesting the food you eat is the primary purpose of stomach acid, so if you eliminate a good portion of your stomach acid, your body is prohibited from or less efficient in its work of digestion. Also, stomach acid is "our first line of defense against pathogens, bacteria, parasites, etc." that enter the body through the mouth.[23]

The result of blocking stomach acid may be temporary relief from heartburn or reflux. But the acid blockers allow the bad bacteria to multiply because stomach acid kills bacteria and lack of stomach acid enables bacteria to flourish. This imbalance is bad news for your gut! An overgrowth of bad bacteria is often the natural result.

The acid in the stomach is not the problem. It is there to help you digest food and to protect you by killing off any harmful microbes before they reach your colon, the last part of your gut. The colon, virtually oxygen free and low in acid, is where most gut bacteria (good and bad) live. The beneficial bacteria in the colon produce short-chain fatty acids, including butyric acid, propionic acid, and acetic acid. Butyric acid fuels the cells lining the colon. The beneficial bacteria also produce vitamin K, vitamin B_{12}, vitamin B_1, and vitamin B_2.

By removing the good and necessary stomach acid, you are allowing the following process:

1. Bad bacteria increase.
2. The bad bacteria may eventually colonize your small intestine, where they do not belong.

3. The bad bacteria can overgrow in the small intestine and cause SIBO, with a lot of bloating, gas, and abdominal pain.

4. Inflammation usually occurs and typically spreads to other parts of your body.

5. Weight gain usually occurs because your stomach acid is needed to break down the protein you eat.[24]

One of the leading causes of IBS is the lack of stomach acid in the gut![25] Another result of knocking out stomach acid is an increased risk of dementia.[26]

And yet another possible side effect of taking antacids is sarcopenia (muscle wasting). This is common with senior citizens who are usually protein deficient—not because they are failing to eat enough proteins but because they have no stomach acid to digest the protein and utilize the foods they are eating! Quite simply, if the protein cannot be broken down into amino acids and used, it passes right through, and you get muscle wasting and sarcopenia.[27]

Your body desperately needs stomach acid, so don't get rid of it. And if you are told you need antacids, find an alternative that addresses the real issues, not one that masks one symptom but then brings with it a host of other problems.

Alternatives/options/choices

Think twice before taking acid-blocking meds and antacids. Thankfully, there are many alternatives these days, such as these:

- aloe vera
- apple cider vinegar
- deglycyrrhizinated licorice (DGL)
- ginger
- mastic gum

These are all available at most health-food stores. Whether you are young or old, it is possible to fix your gut and maximize your health without jeopardizing it by taking acid-blocking drugs and antacids. (Refer to the acid reflux/GERD section in chapter 8 for more information.)

CAUSE 4 OF LEAKY GUT: GMO FOODS

Much can and needs to be said about genetically modified organism (GMO) foods. It is naïve to think that pesticides, insecticides, or herbicides can be added to seeds on the theory that they will pass through the human body without doing any damage while at the same time harming pests or diseases that attack the plant.

Why would anyone willingly swallow any pesticide, insecticide, or herbicide? At all? Ever? And what's more, why would anyone think it would not affect us—our bodies, our brains, our digestion, our gut bacteria—or our children?

GMO foods were not introduced to the US food supply until the 1990s. Approved by the FDA but banned in many other countries, GMO foods include these well-known food crops:

- alfalfa—about 13.5 percent GMO[28]
- canola (for oil)—95 percent GMO[29]
- corn—92 percent GMO[30]
- cotton (used to make cottonseed oil)—94 percent GMO[31]
- papaya—over 90 percent GMO (of those grown in Hawaii)[32]
- soy—94 percent GMO[33]
- sugar beets (used to make granulated sugar)—99.9 percent GMO[34]

As if that is not enough, the common herbicide known as glyphosate is often sprayed on non-GMO crops, such as wheat and other grass crops, right before harvest to increase yield by speeding up the drying process.[35]

Gastrointestinal disorders have been on the rise for the past fifty years, which means GMOs are not the only cause. But GMO foods do play a big part in the gut issues we face today.

It is not a surprise to find that glyphosate—a weed killer—has been found to disrupt the balance of good and bad bacteria in the gut and promote the growth of harmful bacteria.[36] What happens is that the good bacteria, which are necessary for proper digestion, are more easily damaged by glyphosate than the bad bacteria.[37] And that is why the bad bacteria overpopulate while the good bacteria are killed off or struggle to survive. Your health pays the price for losing the bacteria battle.

IT'S A FACT

Digestion is impaired because GMO foods reduce digestive enzymes.[38]

Not only do GMOs increase gut permeability, but they also mess with your immune system, increase infection rates, and negatively affect mood and behavior.[39] They also lower serotonin levels and mess up thyroid hormone production.[40]

Like glyphosate, another herbicide called Bt toxin (found in GMO corn) has been found to damage the gut lining, mimicking the damage done to the gut of those with Celiac disease.[41] Here are a couple more small details about Bt toxin that you should remember:

- Bt toxin in GMO corn "kills insects by punching holes in their digestive tracts, and a 2012 study confirmed that it punctures holes in human cells as well."[42]
- Bt toxin "survives human digestion, and has been detected in the blood of 93% of pregnant women tested and 80% of their unborn fetuses."[43]

These insecticides, herbicides, and pesticides don't just pass through your digestive system. They stick around and cause a lot of damage, including punching holes in your gut wall!

IT'S A FACT

"Eating GM foods alters our genes, . . . triggering our inability [to] burn sugar correctly, making us fatter."[44]

Some in the medical community estimate that about 80 percent of the US population has leaky gut syndrome to some degree.[45] That may be true, but I would say that over 98 percent of my patients suffer from leaky gut, and it is usually more than just a minor irritant. They typically have substantial damage to their gut walls, good bacteria, and digestion.

Leaky gut syndrome plays a primary role in most autoimmune disorders, food sensitivities, IBS, multiple sclerosis (MS), and even some cancers.[46] Anything that contributes to a leaky gut should be minimized and eventually removed from our diet.

You may be thinking, "Well, that's easy. I'll just stop eating GMO foods." That's easier said than done. As we just read, an estimated 92 percent of corn and 94 percent of soy grown in the US are genetically modified.[47] And that means almost all foods with any corn or soy ingredients are GMO. This includes high-fructose corn syrup, the sweetener found in almost all processed foods and drinks in the US.

All told, some estimate that 80 percent of conventional processed food contains GMOs.[48] Clearly, it's time to cut back on processed foods. The fact is, it's always time to do that!

As the food cycle continues, GMO foods (especially corn) are fed to animals. That includes the beef, poultry, and fish industries, and this trickles right back to us in the meat, milk, cheese, eggs, and farm-raised fish we eat.

Alternatives/options/choices

Since GMO foods seem to be everywhere, what are we to do? Thankfully we live in a day and age where we have a lot of other options.

First, go organic as much as possible. Look for a certified organic seal or a non-GMO statement.

Second, don't eat the most common GMO foods, such as corn and soy, unless they are clearly marked as non-GMO. I always tell patients who have gut issues to go gluten-free, but switching to corn is not necessarily an option. Remember, most US corn is GMO. Not all gluten-free foods will be an option. Going gluten-free is important, but so is avoiding GMO foods as much as possible.

It will take a little time to adjust your food-buying habits, so be patient with yourself. Take your time. You don't have to double your food budget or go hungry. Begin the process of avoiding GMO foods. It won't be long before you settle into a rhythm of finding the right foods.

Cause 5 of Leaky Gut: Chlorine

If you have ever owned a goldfish, you know what happens if you put it in a tank of tap water. The chlorine eventually kills the fish, right? But we drink tap water.

Chlorine has been added to water for more than one hundred years. It has done wonders to prevent cholera and typhoid the world over,[49] but that is not all. It can also kill off good bacteria.

No, it is not at the toxic level of antibiotics in the extreme danger to your gut, but chlorine also kills the beneficial bacteria in your GI tract.[50] You get it into your system when you drink it, go swimming, or take a shower. It's even in the steam in the bathroom during a hot shower.

Basically, you find it everywhere, and it is also toxic to your gut.

Alternatives/options/choices

Despite all the benefits that chlorine has brought to countries around the world, we need to do the best we can to minimize our absorption of chlorine and to avoid drinking or cooking with tap water. Here are a few options:

- If you have a chlorine swimming pool, consider converting it to a saltwater pool.
- Consider installing a water filtration system on your entire house.
- Drink bottled water.
- Invest in a water filter for your kitchen that removes chlorine.
- It might seem silly, but if you shorten your shower time and keep the water slightly cooler so there is no steam to inhale, you can reduce your chlorine exposure considerably. Or purchase and install a shower filter.

You may not be able to avoid it altogether, but the less chlorine in and on your body, the better.

Cause 6 of Leaky Gut: Pesticides

Studies have shown that washing produce does not remove all pesticide residues; however, cold-water washing does remove 75–80 percent of pesticide residues.[51] But if the pesticides are in the food as a result of genetic modification, then the only way to avoid these toxins is to not eat the foods that contain pesticides. (Yes, sadly, "some GMO plants have been engineered to produce pesticides themselves.... Other GMO crops have been modified to be herbicide-tolerant."[52])

Glyphosate is one of the primary herbicides used on GMO foods to protect the crops from pests. US farms apply an estimated 287 million pounds of it every year.[53] But over one thousand different pesticides are used in the world, each with its unique properties and effects on its intended source.[54]

IT'S A FACT

"I am now convinced that leaky gut underlies all our disease issues, just as Hippocrates posited."[55]

The most common way pesticides enter your body is from what you eat and drink, but these pesticides are also found in such places as bug sprays, lawn-care products, and even the air during mosquito-spraying season.

Pesticides mess with your gut and do damage by killing some of the good bacteria, which, as you know, means the bad bacteria are more prone to overpopulate. This only adds to the ongoing imbalance of bacteria in your gut, leading to dysbiosis.[56]

Even if pesticides cause minimal damage to your gut bacteria, repeated exposure, even in small doses, can eventually add up. In this case, it is subtracting good bacteria each time. And you need all the good bacteria you can get—and keep.

Alternatives/options/choices

You cannot lock yourself in your house. But you can minimize your interaction with pesticides by watching what you eat, reading ingredients in the sprays you need to use in regular life, and washing fruits and vegetables before eating.

According to the Environmental Working Group (EWG), the top twelve fruits and vegetables with the most pesticides (called the Dirty Dozen) are as follows (from most pesticides to least):[57]

1. strawberries
2. spinach
3. kale
4. nectarines
5. apples
6. grapes
7. peaches
8. cherries
9. pears
10. tomatoes
11. celery
12. potatoes

Strawberries and spinach were found to have the most pesticide residue compared to other foods on the list, yet these are supposed to be some of the healthiest foods! This is not to say that you should not eat these twelve fruits and vegetables. Washing them well with cold water will help, but you can also use a baking soda and water mix, a saltwater soak, or vinegar soak. Peeling will also work if necessary. It's best to choose organic if you regularly eat these foods.

The EWG also has a Clean Fifteen list that names the produce with the lowest amounts of pesticide residues. The 2020 list is as follows:[58]

1. avocados
2. sweet corn (usually GMO)
3. pineapples
4. onions
5. papaya

6. frozen sweet peas

7. eggplants

8. asparagus

9. cauliflower

10. cantaloupes

11. broccoli

12. mushrooms

13. cabbage

14. honeydew melons

15. kiwi

Again, the list does not mean you can and should consume large quantities of these fifteen fruits and vegetables. For example, I heartily agree that avocado is one of the best foods for your body, gut included, but sweet corn? Most corn is GMO and is a starch, so I would not recommend it.

If you have a vegetable garden, fruit trees, and other plants, there are many natural and safe pesticides you can buy or create on your own. Choosing organic foods is the best option for produce unless a food has a thick peel or is on the Clean Fifteen list. With pesticides, awareness is indeed the first step toward change.

CAUSE 7 OF LEAKY GUT: INTESTINAL INFECTIONS

Although this final cause of a leaky gut is one of the top seven reasons, it is not all that common. What puts intestinal infections on the list is the fact that, many times, they lead to IBS and leaky gut. Intestinal infections can be serious, often make a long-term negative impact, and might be deadly.

People usually associate intestinal infections with traveling to a foreign country and eating foods or drinking water that cause diarrhea within twenty-four hours. These travel-related examples, such as amoebic dysentery, are caused by bacteria or parasites, including giardia, Blastocystis, cryptosporidium, and others.

You don't need to travel to developing countries to come in contact with bacteria or parasites that cause intestinal infections. I have had patients get intestinal infections from food poisoning, especially from salmonella. They are common at day care centers and group homes because the cause is not a virus but rather bacteria or parasites. Once they infect the body, they are difficult to get rid of, and multiple people can contract the infection.

A common consequence of intestinal infection is IBS, with symptoms including diarrhea, nausea, abdominal pain, gas, bloating, etc. Another consequence of intestinal infection is excessive amounts of bad bacteria (called dysbiosis) from parasitic or bacterial infections that kill off sufficient numbers of good bacteria, causing the bad bacteria to gain the advantage.

Both IBS and dysbiosis usually lead directly to leaky gut.

Antibiotics are typically prescribed to combat bacterial infection. They may kill the bacteria causing the infection, but the symptoms often persist, which is a clear sign that the infection has damaged the gut wall by killing off a good portion of the good gut bacteria. The bad bacteria levels have usually increased as a result.

IT'S A FACT

"Sometimes, without the good bacteria, the dangerous ones can grow with abandon, producing toxins that damage the bowel lining and trigger inflammation."[59]

Unfortunately, that is not all there is to intestinal infections. A much more serious bacterial infection is *Clostridioides difficile*, or *C. difficile*, or *C. diff.*, for short, in which the colon gets highly inflamed, causing unstoppable diarrhea (sometimes bloody) that may result in death.

According to the Centers for Disease Control and Prevention (CDC), almost five hundred thousand people are diagnosed with *C. difficile* each year. Here is the CDC's exact explanation of what happens (italics added for emphasis):

> *Patients who take antibiotics are most at risk for developing* C. difficile *infections.* More than half of all hospitalized patients will get an antibiotic at some point during their hospital stay, but studies have shown that *30 percent to 50 percent of antibiotics prescribed in hospitals are unnecessary or incorrect.* When a person takes

broad-spectrum antibiotics, beneficial bacteria that are normally present in the human gut and protect against infection *can be suppressed for several weeks to months*. During this time, patients can get sick from *C. difficile* picked up from contaminated surfaces or spread person to person. *Unnecessary antibiotic use and poor infection control* may increase the spread of *C. difficile* within a facility and from facility to facility when infected patients transfer, such as from a hospital to a nursing home.[60]

Those who get *C. difficile* typically have an imbalanced gut.[61] In nursing homes or hospitals, antibiotic overuse is the primary cause. Chemotherapy treatment can also do it. A gut with too much bad bacteria and not enough good bacteria is an ideal place for *C. difficile* to take hold. For older patients, death from *C. difficile* can come quickly, often within thirty days of the diagnosis![62]

About twenty years ago, I had a patient in her seventies who was in the ICU and developed *C. difficile*. "You are going to die," the doctors told her. Statistically speaking, that was the truth.

As soon as she was released from the hospital, she came to see me and asked for help. "I want to live!" she exclaimed.

I put her on as many probiotics as were available back then. Week after week, we blasted her GI tract with probiotics. The race was on to quickly tip the scales and replenish the good bacteria in her gut. And she beat it! She overcame *C. difficile*, and that's no easy feat.

Alternatives/options/choices

Research shows that at least 50 percent of people who travel to developing countries may come down with "traveler's diarrhea," an intestinal infection that causes diarrhea and other GI symptoms.[63] The goal then is to boost the levels of good bacteria in the gut before, during, and after travel.

Probiotics (especially *Lactobacillus rhamnosus* and *Saccharomyces boulardii*) have been found to protect the gut and reduce the severity of intestinal infections.[64] The recommendation is to eat probiotic-rich foods (such as coconut or goat milk yogurt, or kefir) while traveling.[65] That makes total sense.

Even if you have taken antibiotics to combat the intestinal infection, boost your probiotic intake. Studies have found that probiotics significantly reduce the severity of diarrhea in patients who have had antibiotics.[66]

Some argue that the best way to beat *C. difficile* is to stop taking the antibiotics that caused the damage in the first place.[67] Some antibiotics treat *C. difficile*, and if significant gut damage has occurred, the patient may need a lot of concentrated and immediate help, including specific antibiotics, to survive.[68]

With *C. difficile*, probiotics have been proven to help, and I've used them with my patients. In addition to taking probiotics, one powerful and effective method for beating *C. difficile* is fecal transplants (the transferring of stool from a healthy person to the infected person's colon).[69] This is usually in the form of an enema but can also be a series of pills. The results have proven to be astounding for many patients. While other countries allow fecal transplants for the treatment of a variety of gut-related sicknesses and diseases, here in the US, the FDA allows the use of fecal transplants only to treat *C. difficile*.

The best way to treat intestinal infections is also the best way to live life, and that is with high levels of good bacteria in your gut. Intestinal infections can also lead to small intestinal bacterial overgrowth (SIBO) and small intestinal fungal overgrowth (SIFO), which are discussed in chapter 8.

PART II
GUT DISEASES

Part 2 begins with the gut being at a disadvantage. From this state of increased intestinal permeability, enemies (both expected and unexpected) come out in force. And after they have caused their damage, sickness and disease usually follow.

CHAPTER FIVE

AFTER THE GUT STARTS TO LEAK

Bａｃｋ ｉｎ ｔｈｅ mid-1990s, our family had a ski boat and a lake house on Lake Mary in Lake Mary, Florida. On weekends, we would often go water-skiing. My son, a teenager at the time, had purchased a wakeboard, and one weekend I decided it was time for me to conquer that wakeboard. I tried for over an hour to get up but couldn't do it. I weighed about 220 at the time, and the boat's motor was not strong enough to pull me out of the water, so a lot of dragging and swallowing lake water were going on. It felt like I drank a gallon of lake water before I called it quits!

About two weeks later, I began to experience diarrhea, along with some bloating and gas. It would come and go for several weeks. Finally, I did a parasite test. Sure enough, I had giardia. A parasitic infection is another intestinal infection that damages the GI tract and causes leaky gut.

I promptly took an antibiotic (metronidazole) to kill the parasite, but my IBS (which I already had) took a turn for the worse. The giardia and antibiotics both aggravated my IBS and created a whole new level of inflammation in my gut. If I hadn't had a full-blown leaky gut before, I certainly did at that point.

The damage to my gut was done. Normal foods suddenly caused inflammation in my body. Foods containing tomatoes, peppers, gluten, and dairy were out because the reaction was almost immediate.

It took me years to find all the answers to my IBS, leaky gut, and food issues. Along the way, I discovered (from painful personal experience) that some foods will perpetually keep a damaged gut in a leaky gut state. The foods did not create the problem, but once the leaky gut got a foothold in my body, the once-healthy foods sent waves of damaging inflammation throughout my body.

Once the gut wall becomes more permeable, many foods can damage not only the gut but the whole body as well. Autoimmune diseases can be turned on, and food sensitivities and gut symptoms usually increase. Also, brain issues such as brain fog, memory issues, and a whole lot more symptoms typically develop—all because inflammation in the gut is worsened by food sensitivities.

WHY GOOD FOOD CAN MAKE YOU FEEL BAD

If your gut is out of balance (with more bad bacteria than good) and you have leaky gut but are not suffering from a diagnosed disease, then you may be experiencing some of these symptoms:

- bloating
- brain fog
- constipation
- depression
- diarrhea
- fatigue
- gas
- headache
- heartburn
- itching
- joint pain
- rashes
- short-term memory loss
- stomachache

These symptoms are linked to having a food sensitivity or food intolerance, as some call it. You may have been able to eat a particular food before without any symptoms, but now it causes inflammation and some of the other symptoms listed above.

Usually the symptoms start as mild but get worse. And because an estimated 70–80 percent of your immune system is housed in your GI tract,[1] affecting and impairing your immune system may be the natural next step.

If your gut does not like what you are feeding it, these symptoms are an obvious sign that you need to stop. However, the typical response is to get a prescription. That approach usually improves the symptoms only temporarily, and it does nothing to treat the core problem.

If you cover up food sensitivity symptoms, which are often the result of an already leaking gut, then you are eventually opening yourself up to more medical problems. This is the perfect feeding ground for autoimmune diseases and brain-related issues, such as brain fog, and long term may lead to dementia, Alzheimer's disease, Parkinson's, and much more.

It sounds scary because it is! Inflammation, as seen with the previously listed symptoms, is like a flashing neon sign that says we need to pause and figure out what is wrong. Pretending there is no problem is about as good as covering the symptom with a prescription. Either way, the gut needs help, and if you don't get help, things will most likely get worse.

If the gut is healthy, it's not likely that inflammation will occur. It's usually when the gut is damaged and inflamed with leaky gut and bacterial imbalance (when the bad bacteria outnumber the good) that food sensitivities become serious issues.

Food Allergies

Food sensitivities are usually temporary, superficial, and non-life-threatening. They are usually cleared up by avoiding the food for a period of time and then rotating eating that food every three to seven days in limited amounts until symptoms resolve and following the Healthy Gut Zone diet in chapters 11 and 12. One should also avoid the ten common enemies of the gut in chapter 6. Food allergies, on the other hand, can be painful, long-lasting, and sometimes fatal. Here is a brief list of food allergy symptoms that I have seen:

- acne
- anaphylaxis
- asthma
- bloating/excess weight
- brain fog
- canker sores
- coughing
- dark circles under eyes

- dizziness
- earaches
- eczema/rashes
- fatigue
- headaches/migraines
- hives/urticaria
- mood swings (anxiety, aggressiveness, irritability)
- shortness of breath
- sinus problems
- skin redness
- tight/hoarse throat
- tongue swelling
- vomiting
- weak pulse[2]

With food allergies, we usually learn to avoid offending foods. With food sensitivities, we are much more likely to try to mask the symptoms with medication. But as you know, covering up inflammation will often only make things worse in the long run.

The best answer is always to figure out what causes the problem and stop eating it. For example, if you are allergic to one of the following eight top food allergens, then you have probably already revised your eating habits to avoid it:

1. cow's milk

2. eggs

3. nuts (from trees)

4. peanuts (which are actually legumes, not nuts)

5. shellfish

6. wheat

7. soy

8. fish[3]

Typically, if you are allergic to these foods and inadvertently eat them, you will suddenly develop one or more of the previously listed symptoms. An immune system reaction is triggered, producing antibodies called immunoglobulin E (IgE), which travel to your cells and release chemicals that create the symptoms of an allergic reaction.

IT'S A FACT

People with autoimmune diseases usually have high zonulin levels and a leaky gut.[4]

You must understand that if you have a leaky gut, foods you are not allergic to but are sensitive to can create a similar immune response, but your symptoms will be delayed by hours or even days and not occur immediately like a true food allergy. Typically, food sensitivities or intolerances are not sudden or severe and are mediated with higher levels of IgG, IgA, and IgM, not IgE. You will probably not experience shortness of breath, hives, dizziness, anaphylaxis, or tongue swelling, but know your gut is waging the battle. That is because these foods, at the molecular level, are causing inflammation, which usually worsens a leaky gut, increases your bad bacteria, and decreases your beneficial bacteria.

If you suddenly couldn't breathe after eating a particular food, you would naturally quit eating it, right? But because the battle is being waged down in the gut and may occur hours or days after eating the offending food or foods, the tendency is to keep right on eating the offending foods. Most people don't realize that certain foods are causing more inflammation in the gut because the symptoms don't occur immediately but are delayed. The Healthy Gut Zone diet removes most foods that trigger food sensitivities.

Can You Measure Leaky Gut?

How leaky is your gut? Is it leaking at all? Odds are, I have found that most of my patients have leaky gut to some degree. If you have some of the symptoms we have discussed so far, especially those of an autoimmune disease, then it is virtually guaranteed that you have a leaky gut.

When we have a leaky gut, does the severity level matter? Yes. It can matter, and thankfully it is now possible to measure the degree of a leaky gut we have.

With most of my patients, we simply assume (because they are sick, have symptoms, and know their track record) they have leaky gut. That is often the best approach. But tests can be done (usually blood tests) to measure the severity of damage to the gut wall. Several markers measure whether or not you have a leaky gut.

One measurable marker is zonulin, which was discovered in 2000 by Dr. Alessio Fasano, a gastroenterologist at the University of Maryland School of Medicine. Zonulin is a protein that plays a role in managing the permeability of the gut. The higher the amount of zonulin in your blood, the greater the intestinal permeability of your gut wall. The zonulin proteins increase for two main reasons: (1) bad bacteria in the gut and (2) gluten in the foods we eat.[5]

Besides serum zonulin testing, other tests to measure leaky gut or increased intestinal permeability include these:

- differential sugar test with lactulose and mannitol
- antibody testing
  - « zonulin-occludin antibodies
  - « actomyosin antibodies
  - « antibodies to LPS (lipopolysaccharides)

The test that I usually do for a leaky gut is the Cyrex Array 2 Intestinal Antigenic Permeability screen, which measures actomyosin IgG, occludin/zonulin IgG, occludin/zonulin IgA, occludin/zonulin IgM, LPS IgG, LPS IgA, and LPS IgM.

As we noted, interestingly, gluten shows up as a common cause for increased zonulin levels. The next chapter outlines the top ten common enemies to your gut, and it just so happens that gluten is the number one enemy! But once the gut has been damaged, there are a lot more enemies than you may have imagined.

CHAPTER SIX

TEN COMMON ENEMIES OF YOUR GUT

WHEN YOU HAVE severe leaky gut and too much bad bacteria in your GI tract, you will usually find very few foods that don't inflame your gut. The temptation is to eat only these few things, but that is not a healthy long-term option.

I had a patient several years ago who had reduced her diet down to water and a handful of solid foods. "Everything else makes my gut ache and bloat," she complained. "So, I basically quit eating."

She had pushed her body so far that she had multiple lists of symptoms. At first glance, there was no one single problem. Almost everything caused inflammation, and that inflammation was being expressed in the form of several inflammatory and autoimmune diseases, including osteoarthritis, eczema, psoriasis, GERD, Hashimoto's thyroiditis, fibromyalgia, and chronic fatigue.

For her, eating food that provided her gut with the nutrients she needed gave her more options than she was currently allowed to enjoy. But it was the Healthy Gut Zone diet, along with probiotics, prebiotics, fiber, and a handful of select supplements, that helped begin to turn the tide in her gut.

Due to the severity of her condition, we ran several tests to see how bad her leaky gut was. Her gut was leaking like a sieve, and as you would expect, her immune system was equally as messed up, which explained why she had so many ailments going on at once.

The good news is that she pulled through just fine. She stuck to the regimen, and her body responded amazingly well to what we did to restore her gut. A mere twelve months later, you would not have recognized her! Her complexion, skin color, dull eyes, dark rings under her eyes, saggy skin, and positive attitude were significantly improved. Her joint pain disappeared, her skin cleared up, her muscle aches left, her energy improved dramatically, and her brain fog lifted. Her list of meds went from five down to zero, and this was especially good news because two of her medications (Celebrex and Nexium) had contributed to her leaky gut.

She no longer suffered from those previously diagnosed diseases. Her immune system no longer struggled to keep her body healthy, she no longer had a leaky gut, and she no longer lived on a diet that would have made a prisoner revolt. It was all in her gut. When she fixed that, it restored her health, and she was back on top of the world.

COMMON ENEMIES COME FROM INSIDE

Leaky gut (often called increased intestinal permeability) and excessive bad bacteria (dysbiosis) set the stage for a limitless number of problems. These problems come from the inside, usually as a reaction to foods and medications. To make matters worse, many of the offending foods were once your friends—or at least were neutral—before they became your enemies.

Some argue that you should go on an elimination diet, but that will be truly helpful only *after* you have restored your gut. Until that point, you will get false readings for the following reasons:

- Bad bacteria are usually in control. Too much bad bacteria can result in inflammation, leaky gut, and immune reactions.
- The gut wall is leaking. Gaps between gut wall cells allow large particles to enter the bloodstream, which triggers inflammation or food sensitivity reactions.[1]

As soon as you have a leaky gut, other food sensitivities generally appear, but that is not all. Inflammation, a weakened immune system, and an increased risk for sickness and disease follow right behind.[2] This is why it is so vital that you regain control in your gut.

Usually, when the good bacteria are in control and the gut wall has healed, the inflammation subsides, symptoms disappear, and food sensitivities decrease. That is also when diseases will be able to fade away.

Until that point, you will have to put up with ten common enemies. If you have an unhealthy gut, these are usually the ten most common enemies your gut will be fighting:

1. gluten

2. a high-sugar, high-carb diet

3. dairy

4. lectins

5. artificial sweeteners

6. emulsifiers

7. saturated fats

8. constipation

9. stress

10. staying too clean

You might find that the following descriptions and symptoms of the ten common enemies apply to you and your situation. If so, that is completely normal. The next step then is to find the root cause and fix it. You will also need to avoid GMO foods (discussed in chapter 4), including most corn, soy, canola oil, cottonseed oil, and sugar beets. Only by doing these things can your gut be restored. And a healthy gut is a requirement for good health.

COMMON ENEMY 1: GLUTEN

The most common enemy to your gut, especially *after* your gut has been compromised (with too much bad bacteria and leaky gut) but often even *before* it is compromised, is gluten. It is probably the most dangerous enemy to your gut health as well.

Gluten is the protein found in wheat, barley, and rye, as well as all the bread, pasta, bagels, pretzels, cereals, cakes, cookies, and processed foods made with these gluten-rich flours. An enemy that can negatively affect you both before and after leaky gut is bad enough, but the impact of gluten can be severe, wide-reaching, and long-term.

Did you know the following facts?

- For *some*, gluten sets off an autoimmune reaction that can destroy the villi of the small intestine. These patients have celiac disease.

- For *many*, gluten is a food sensitivity.

- For *everyone* who has an unhealthy gut, gluten causes a *lot* of problems!

Here is another thought: today's common wheat can produce 23,788 different proteins, and any of them have the potential of triggering inflammation.[3] Since wheat has that many different proteins, it might be best if you avoid it. I recommend this, especially if your gut has been compromised.

However, most inflammation and damage are usually caused by two specific gluten proteins: glutenins and gliadins. People are often sensitive to one or both of these proteins.[4] The typical symptoms of gluten sensitivity include the following:

- abdominal pain
- bloating and gas
- constipation
- diarrhea
- fatigue
- nausea
- numbness in legs, arms, or fingers[5]

A gliadin sensitivity can be especially damaging to your body because it increases gut permeability (leaky gut) in *everyone*,[6] and it triggers a release of brain-assaulting inflammation.[7]

IT'S A FACT

"It's possible for virtually **everyone** *to have a negative, albeit undetected, reaction" to gluten, which in turn causes lasting damage without one even knowing it.*[8]

A weakened gut can lead to a leaky brain,[9] and you do not even need to be diagnosed with celiac disease for this to be true. If your gut is not healthy, there is a very big chance that gliadin is causing inflammation somewhere in your body!

Some argue that everyone is gliadin sensitive, whether they have a healthy gut or not. That may be the case. I would say that if your gut is healthy and your gluten intake is minimal, you are probably fine. But if your gut is not healthy, then I would recommend that you go gluten-free for at least six months to a full year. At a later date, after your gut has healed itself, you might be able to consume small and occasional amounts of gluten foods, but until then, you should avoid gluten altogether.

IT'S A FACT

White Bread vs. Brown Bread

We used to say, "The whiter your bread, the sooner you're dead." But that is not the case! White bread has gluten, but whole wheat bread has gluten and wheat germ agglutinin (WGA). This small WGA protein passes easily through your gut wall, and it causes weight gain, results in insulin resistance, impairs digestion of protein, causes inflammation, crosses the blood/brain barrier, may cause neurological problems, and more. Avoid bran and whole grain. In short, browner bread varieties are worse for your gut than whiter bread varieties.[10]

Gluten (gliadin specifically) is bad for you because gliadin triggers an excessive release of zonulin, which causes the tight junctions between the intestinal cells to open wider, producing a leaky gut. As we have discussed, zonulin is a protein in charge of opening and closing the tiny barriers in the gut wall. So the more zonulin release you have, the more inflammation and potential for an autoimmune response you will have as a direct result.[11]

Dr. David Perlmutter describes gluten as a "silent germ" because it secretly causes a lot of damage without your being aware of it.[12] This fact comes into play when the damage to the gut continues for years and years without a break. When the gut ends up more inflamed and with a greater degree of being leaky, that can eventually lead to autoimmune diseases such as Crohn's disease, ulcerative colitis, multiple sclerosis, type 1 diabetes, lupus, rheumatoid arthritis, vasculitis, alopecia areata, polymyalgia rheumatica, Raynaud's disease, vitiligo, thyroiditis, and Sjögren's syndrome.[13]

There are countless more ailments and diseases to add to that list, such as depression, dementia, Alzheimer's, Parkinson's, and more. Having your body attack itself leads to so many diseases and symptoms!

Alternatives/options/choices

Unfortunately, gluten is everywhere, even in places where you would not expect it. Since the 1950s, commercial bakers in the US have used transglutaminase (also called vital gluten), rather than the traditional yeast, to make the bread rise.[14] The reason is that it creates a better texture, increases chewiness, and extends shelf life.[15]

IT'S A FACT

"Changes in your gut's environment can undermine the brain's ability to protect itself against potentially toxic invaders."[16]

Using plain old yeast is best because it ferments and destroys much of the gluten, lectins, and sugar. That is why sourdough bread is not as bad for you. I go gluten-free myself because I am gluten sensitive, but when I am in Europe, I can usually eat their bread without incident. Why? Because they still use yeast, while much of our bread here in the US uses vital gluten. The difference can be felt immediately in your gut.

But transglutaminase, FDA approved to be used by US commercial bakers, does not destroy the gluten, lectins, or sugars. It crosses the blood/brain barrier and causes damage. Transglutaminase actually increases sensitivity to gluten.[17]

But that is not all. Transglutaminase is also added to processed meats as a food additive to bind water and fats.[18] It works as a "meat glue" to hold the meat together.

In other words, gluten is not only in all the typical bready places; it is also in ground meats, such as hamburger meat and ground beef. If you are trying to avoid gluten, you will need to do your homework. The peak awareness in today's society about gluten does make it easier than ever to do the necessary research and to avoid gluten. (See appendix C for an extensive list of food items that do or may contain gluten.)

What you eat helps control your inflammation, balances your blood sugar levels, and affects your gut and gut bacteria.[19] So watch what you eat, and limit or eliminate gluten. Your body will directly benefit as a result.

COMMON ENEMY 2: A HIGH-SUGAR, HIGH-CARB DIET

The second-greatest cause of inflammation and increased leaky gut that I see is a high-sugar, high-carb diet. It makes sense when you think about it because bacteria usually grow unchecked in a sugary environment. Naturally, it is not the good bacteria that are growing in the gut of someone who eats high-sugar, high-carb foods.

Keep in mind that the standard diet in North America is not only high in sugar and carbs but also low in fiber. That means increased inflammation, gut wall damage, immune system damage, and a host of illnesses with their corresponding symptoms. It is a cycle of more bacteria growth that leads to increased inflammation, followed by more growth, etc.[20] If left unchecked, conditions will likely only get worse.

The International Foundation for Gastrointestinal Disorders estimates that 10–15 percent of the worldwide population has IBS.[21] ADHD diagnoses are on the rise, along with depression, anxiety, autoimmune disease, cardiovascular disease, and the much-feared dementia and Alzheimer's disease. All of these are attached to a leaky gut!

Ideally you want your gut to be healthy and not be home to inflammation. That, in turn, is good for every part of your body, including your brain.

IT'S A FACT

Until the gut is healthy, our bodies almost always crave the foods that cause the most damage, which are usually sugar and carbs.

What people may not know about carbohydrates is that they spike blood sugar levels. High blood sugar levels help throw the body's bacteria levels out of balance and fuel inflammation.[22] This imbalance leads to increased food sensitivities and more inflammation, always worsening the current situation, little by little.

Alternatives/options/choices

We can (and should) eat foods that help to control inflammation and keep our good bacteria levels high. We can do that by keeping the blood sugar levels low. That means not eating what everyone else is eating. High-sugar, high-carb diets will not help anyone live a healthy life.

The best diet to balance bacteria levels and decrease inflammation is one that is low in carbohydrates. But you don't want to cut out all carbs completely. For the long term, I suggest not going lower than 50 grams of carbs per day. If you go lower than that long term, you can harm your gut and hurt your good bacteria.[23] If you are getting enough fiber (such as psyllium husk powder), then you could go low (25 grams of carbs a day for women, 35 grams of carbs a day for men) without harming yourself.

Your body always needs a small to moderate amount of proteins (meats that are organic or grass-fed, ideally), lots of vegetables (to feed your good bacteria), and plenty of fiber.

Talking of food recommendations and carbohydrates, consider resistant starches. These low-sugar, healthy carbs remain undigested until they reach your colon. At that point, they ferment to produce short-chain fatty acids, which are tremendously beneficial for your gut.[24]

Three great examples of resistant starches are green bananas, green mangoes, and green papayas. They provide you with healthy carbs, and in their green state, they are very low in sugar. We will talk more about resistant starches later, along with other specific foods that feed the good bacteria in your gut. With so many options today, there is no reason that anyone would settle for a high-sugar, high-carbohydrate diet.

Carbohydrates and starches to avoid or curb include wheat, corn, rice, oats, all grains, potatoes, beans, peas, lentils, and fruit. We need to avoid sugary foods and consume only about 50–100 grams of healthy carbs a day, which we will discuss in part 3 of this book.

COMMON ENEMY 3: DAIRY

It is no surprise that dairy is on the list of the most common enemies of your gut. It regularly ranks as one of the top items to which people are allergic or sensitive. In fact, cow's milk is the number one food allergen of people around the world.

The sugar in milk (lactose) causes the digestive problems known as lactose intolerance in many people. It may cause inflammation, which is not beneficial for the gut or the rest of the body. If someone is lactose intolerant, he or she cannot digest the lactose in milk or milk products.

IT'S A FACT

Symptoms of lactose intolerance include bloating, gas, diarrhea, abdominal pain, rumbling sounds, and nausea.

Also, because lactose is a sugar, it affects gut bacteria similarly to the number two common enemy: a high-sugar, high-carbohydrate diet. The sugar in the gut boosts the bad bacteria and adds to the overall inflammation in the gut.

For people who are working to restore their guts to healthy levels, I strongly recommend going dairy free for a minimum of several months as their guts clear up. This will give enough time for their good gut bacteria to be replenished and their gut inflammation to be decreased. Whether lactose intolerant or not, it has been found that most people will feel better when they eliminate dairy from their diet.[25]

Alternatives/options/choices

We have known for years that many dairy-sensitive people can consume milk, cheese, and yogurt from sheep or goats. It's dairy products from cows that they have to avoid. But not all milk is created equal. There are two distinct types of cow's milk, and the second is becoming increasingly popular these days. If you have thought you were lactose intolerant or dairy sensitive, this might mean more dairy choices for you.

Milk that comes from Holstein (also called Friesian), Ayrshire, and Milking Shorthorn cows usually contains both A1 beta-casein and A2 beta-casein. But Guernsey, Jersey, Charolais, and Limousin cows have a genetic mutation that results in their milk protein having only A2 beta-casein.[26]

IT'S A FACT

If you have gut issues when you eat certain foods, stop eating them for a while. When the gut is healed and inflammation is turned down or off, then you can eat them every three to four days or perhaps more often. This is true for food sensitives, but food allergies will usually remain with you for life.

It turns out that some people who think they are lactose intolerant (unable to digest the milk sugar) might actually have trouble digesting one of the *proteins* (A1 beta-casein) rather than the *sugar* (lactose) in the milk. These people are not lactose intolerant but are still dairy sensitive. The good news is that dairy-sensitive people may be able to enjoy A2 dairy products without the same digestive reaction and inflammation that they have with regular dairy.[27]

It's exciting to think that people who thought they needed to avoid milk might have new options, but it's important to remember that all milk still contains sugar. So if you are trying to balance the good bacteria in your gut, going without dairy for a season will probably still be necessary.

If you are lactose intolerant and choose to consume dairy, you can add lactase enzyme drops just before you consume dairy or limit your dairy intake to two to four ounces at a time.

COMMON ENEMY 4: LECTINS

This common enemy of your gut may not be all that well known, but it is a major player in causing inflammation and leaky gut. The name of this common enemy is lectins.

Lectins were first discovered in 1888 and were later used in research of blood type differences.[28] According to some, lectins are likely to be found in around 30–40 percent of the foods we typically eat in the American diet. They are primarily concentrated in grains (especially wheat), seeds, nuts, legumes (especially soy), nightshade plants (potatoes, tomatoes, eggplant, peppers, etc.), and dairy.[29]

Lectins are proteins that plants use as a self-defense mechanism against predators. If a plant is allowed to ripen before harvesting, it naturally reduces the number of lectins. But our modern food system causes us to harvest plants early so they can be transported to grocery stores across the country without going bad. In doing this, these foods are harvested when their lectins are still at peak levels, and the lectin-induced digestive discomforts an animal or other predator would receive from eating that plant in the wild before it was ripe are the same ones we experience when we eat the plant that has been harvested too early.[30] A few common lectin-related symptoms are bloating, diarrhea, fatigue, heartburn, inflammation, nausea, and vomiting.[31]

IT'S A FACT

The most-famous lectin is gluten.

If you feel bad after you have eaten something, it could very well be your body reacting to the lectins. Weight gain, bloating, gas, and brain fog are often lectins working against you. Gluten is the most famous lectin, but did you know that the poison ricin (from a castor bean) is deadly because of its high lectin count?[32] So if you start to think of lectins as poisons, you are right.

What exactly do lectins do to your gut? They attach to your gut wall and pull the cells of your gut wall apart! In addition to directly causing leaky gut, they also disrupt communicating with your immune system, which creates even more bad news for your body.[33] After the lectins go to work in your GI tract, you naturally feel bad and eventually may begin to develop symptoms and autoimmune issues as if you were food poisoned.[34]

Nobody wants to be poisoned, but lectins are mini poison bombs. At the chemical level, it's a battle, and since lectins are not digested, their presence may eventually cause an autoimmune defense response. The good microbes in your gut fight against things that can cause harm, and that is why they fight against the lectins in the first place.[35]

Most food sensitivities may be immune responses to the lectins we consume.[36]

Your body's layers of defense against lectins (nasal mucus, saliva, stomach acid, bacteria in your mouth and gut, and mucus of your gut wall) do their best.[37] But lectins are not digested, and with constant lectin intake and an already leaky gut, it is too much for your body to handle. The autoimmune response is a natural next step, and that means the following may develop:

- altered gut flora
- cellular death
- decreased cellular repair
- disease
- inflammation
- intestinal damage
- malabsorption[38]

Alternatives/options/choices

Nobody wants anything like food poisoning, and thus we should avoid lectins, especially if we have a leaky gut. But what does that mean on a practical level? What foods can we eat or not eat? And are there any other options?

Talking about lectins, if patients are working to restore their gut health, then they need to take a little more drastic action than someone who already has restored his or her gut. That may require some food changes.

The foods with a lot of lectins that I tell patients to avoid also usually happen to be GMO foods and foods full of gluten. The top four lectin foods to *avoid* when you are getting your gut back into shape are as follows:

1. wheat

2. corn

3. meats (beef, chicken, or fish) if fed corn or wheat

4. beans, peas, and lentils (including peanuts, which are
   legumes, and all soy products, which are usually GMO)

Meats that are grass fed or pasture raised and grass or pasture finished are fine to eat, as they were not fed a diet of corn, soy, or wheat. Similarly, the milk and cheese from these grass-fed animals are much lower in lectins and safer to eat.

If you are working on getting your gut back into shape, here are more lectin foods that you will want to minimize or avoid:

- dairy (limited amounts of A2 dairy products are allowed but
  not recommended)

- nightshades (tomatoes, eggplant, potatoes, paprika, goji berries, and peppers—including jalapeno, bell pepper, and cayenne but not black pepper)

- other grains (barley, rye, oats, rice [especially brown rice],
  and quinoa, which are all high in lectins). Millet and sorghum are the only grains that contain no lectins.[39] Indian white basmati rice is lower in lectins than other rice varieties but should be pressure-cooked.

- seed fruits (squash, zucchini, cucumbers, pumpkin)

With legumes, soaking for twenty-four hours, discarding the water before cooking, and pressure-cooking (see the sidebar on this page) will do wonders to break down virtually all lectins. I have seen drastic differences in patients who pressure-cook their legumes as compared to those who do not. Try it yourself to see if you can feel the difference.

With seed fruits and nightshades, removing the seeds and skins will instantly remove almost all the lectins. The lectins hide there, especially in the seeds, so if you throw out the seeds and skins, the pulp or fruit that remains is usually fine to eat. This is very important, especially with tomatoes and peppers.

IT'S A FACT

Reducing Lectins in Beans

Soaking dry legumes, discarding the water, and then cooking with a pressure cooker (just seven and a half minutes) will remove almost all the lectins. Functional medicine practitioner Jordan Reasoner has a specific process for soaking. He uses four cups of water per cup of beans. After soaking the beans and discarding the water, rinse, and then cook.

Black beans, garbanzo beans: soak eighteen to twenty-four hours, adding two tablespoons lemon juice or vinegar per cup of beans.

Lentils, fava beans: soak ten hours, adding two tablespoons lemon juice or vinegar per cup of beans.

Dried and split peas: soak ten hours, adding one pinch of baking soda per cup of beans.

Kidney and cannellini beans: soak eighteen to twenty-four hours in plain water.[40]

I have seen autoimmune diseases like lupus, rheumatoid arthritis, Hashimoto's thyroiditis, Crohn's, and others reverse completely or improve in patients who stopped eating the foods that caused their bodies to react. The body can usually heal when you take out the offending foods.

One patient suffering for ten years from rheumatoid arthritis was taking her prescriptions and doing pretty well. She had no joint pain, stiffness, or deformities. When I asked if she wanted to eventually wean off her medications by first removing the foods that caused the inflammation, she declined. Why? Because the primary lectin-rich food that she would have to give up was tomatoes, and she loved them! She had a leaky gut but refused to quit eating tomatoes, the inflammatory food that was giving her so much trouble. Now, if she peeled and deseeded her tomatoes, that would remove the majority of lectins. It would have been a small price to pay for her health, but she didn't want to go to that much trouble.

IT'S A FACT

If you have IBS or Crohn's, your gut lining is extra sensitive to lectins.[41]

Years ago (before I realized what I was doing), I used to eat a yummy Mexican lunch. Five days a week, I ate salsa with corn chips and then drank the salsa juice. I figured the fresh tomatoes and peppers were healthy because tomatoes are high in the phytonutrient lycopene.

I already had IBS at the time, and my daily routine was wreaking even more havoc on my gut. Strange as it sounds, I craved the very food that was burning holes in my gut! When I stopped eating this gut-inflaming food for lunch, a short three months later, my psoriasis cleared up! Yes, I had already gone gluten-free, but removing the lectins in the form of peppers and tomatoes (typical nightshades) was a necessary part of my gut's healing process.

Today, I can eat a little gluten and modest amounts of tomatoes and peppers, but I know my gut is happier when my diet is low in gluten and low in lectins (especially tomatoes and peppers). I have found that Indian white basmati rice and organic non-GMO corn don't cause inflammation in my gut. I can occasionally have some sourdough bread, as the fermenting process destroys most of the gluten and wheat germ agglutinins.

Most likely, based on hundreds of patients who have worked to restore their gut health, your gut will also improve when you back off (or stop completely) gluten and lectins. Try it. You may like how you feel so much that you will never want to go back!

IT'S A FACT

White flour has fewer lectins than wheat flour, which makes healthy white bread (i.e., sourdough) a viable option (in moderation) when your gut is healed.

Once your gut has been repaired and you properly cook foods that have lectins, you will probably be fine eating those foods again. However, if you have an autoimmune disease, you may need to stay off lectins completely; be extra careful and eat only small amounts; or pressure-cook your beans, peas, and lentils and peel and deseed your tomatoes and peppers.

The goal, of course, is to get your gut healed first.

COMMON ENEMY 5: ARTIFICIAL SWEETENERS

The next common enemy to your gut, gut wall, and overall health is artificial sweeteners. These fake sugars or noncaloric artificial sweeteners (NAS) have been recognized as bad for your health for years. Just how bad and what they do to your body are becoming more evident as time goes by.

Here are common artificial sweeteners to avoid absolutely:

- acesulfame potassium (brand names: Sunett, Sweet One, Sweet & Safe)
- alitame (brand name: Aclame)
- aspartame (brand names: NutraSweet, Equal, Spoonful, Equal-Measure, Canderel, Benevia, AminoSweet, NatraTaste)
- aspartame-acesulfame salt (brand name: Twinsweet)
- cyclamate (brand names: Sucaryl, Cologran)
- saccharin (brand names: Sweet'N Low, Necta Sweet, Cologran, Heremesetas, Sucaryl, Sucron, Sugar Twin, Sweet 10)
- sucralose (brand names: Splenda, Nevella)[42]

IT'S A FACT

Fake sugars make you gain weight.[43]

Perhaps you grew up using artificial sweeteners or have gotten into the habit of not checking the ingredients on what is in your refrigerator or pantry. This is very common, but you may want to reconsider after reading the following lists of reactions to just two artificial sweeteners.

Aspartame reaction list

- abdominal cramps/pain
- change in heart rate
- change in mood
- change in vision
- convulsions and seizures
- diarrhea
- dizziness/poor equilibrium
- fatigue and weakness
- hallucination
- headache
- hives
- joint pain
- memory loss
- nausea and vomiting
- rash
- sleep problems/insomnia[44]

Sucralose reaction list

- allergic reactions
- blood sugar increases
- blurred vision
- dizziness
- gastrointestinal problems
- migraines
- seizures
- weight gain[45]

Due to their chemical properties, some artificial sweeteners can make it all the way to the colon, where they ferment and usually cause bloating and gas.[46] The artificial sweeteners listed above also damage your gut microbiome by helping to kill off your good bacteria and promoting the growth of bad bacteria. According to the international journal *Nature*, artificial sweeteners have been linked directly to dysbiosis and metabolic abnormalities.[47]

IT'S A FACT

"Fructose goes right to the liver and triggers lipogenesis (fat accumulation in the liver), which causes liver damage to 70 million people around the world annually."[48]

The above lists are further proof of the negative impact artificial sweeteners have on the gut. Unfortunately, a sweetener doesn't have to be unnatural to be bad for your gut. You already know how common enemy number 2 (high-sugar, high-carb diets) affects the body. Fruit sugar, or fructose, is another sugar that feeds the bad bacteria in the gut. Fructose causes visceral fat—the most dangerous type of body fat to have—to accumulate around your organs. It is linked to health issues like diabetes, heart disease, and fatty liver.[49]

Another unfortunate trait about fructose and artificial sweeteners is that they do not stimulate insulin production like regular sugar (glucose) does. What that means is that leptin, which tells your body you are full, is *not* released into your body or your brain, and that leaves you still feeling hungry.[50] This is the main reason why artificial sweeteners cause you to gain even more weight than sugar does. They make you hungrier and craving even more sugary foods!

IT'S A FACT

High-fructose corn syrup (HFCS) is a sweetener made from corn syrup. But did you know these facts about it?

» *Ketchup, barbecue sauce, and even salad dressing often contain HFCS.*

» *HFCS comprises 40 percent of caloric sweeteners added to foods and beverages.*

> » *HFCS is the only caloric sweetener in soft drinks in the United States.*[51]

You guessed it: artificial sweeteners, including the natural fructose, are bad for your gut and bad for your metabolism.

Alternatives/options/choices

My opinion on sweeteners is, if you can, to train your body to not need much of them, especially with drinks such as coffee or tea. Many patients practice using less and less in their drinks until they no longer need sweeteners at all.

If you do need sweeteners in baking or in your coffee or tea, I suggest the natural sweeteners such as stevia, erythritol, or monk fruit (lo han guo). Even better is to use chicory root natural sweeteners such as inulin, which is a prebiotic and does not raise blood glucose levels. Just Like Sugar is a natural sweetener made from chicory root. Try stevia with your coffee and tea as well.

The bottom line is that both artificial sweeteners and sugar promote the growth of bad bacteria and kill off your good bacteria, which leads to dysbiosis and leaky gut. To heal your gut, you must eliminate both artificial sweeteners and sugars.

COMMON ENEMY 6: EMULSIFIERS

The next common enemy has a strange name: emulsifier. What is that? The best way to describe an emulsifier is to think of it as a chemical that allows you to mix two different liquids. Or to say it another way: "Emulsifiers are detergent-like molecules that help mix two liquids that don't easily mix, like oil and water."[52]

Oil and water naturally separate from each other, but with an emulsifier added, the two ingredients can be mixed and stay mixed. You will often find emulsifiers in the following:

- baked goods
- candy
- ice cream
- mayonnaise

- processed meats
- salad dressings
- sauces

Emulsifiers offer many more options for food ingredients, consistency, smoothness, shelf life, and visual appeal.

As you can imagine, these "detergent-like molecules" do real damage to your gut, gut wall, and good bacteria.[53] And as with artificial sweeteners, these emulsifiers also mess up your appetite control hormones. They actually make you hungrier![54]

Alternatives/options/choices

There are two primary ways to decrease your intake of emulsifiers:

1. Try to avoid eating foods that contain emulsifiers. Processed foods are the primary source.

2. Make your own foods, such as salad dressings, naturally and without emulsifiers. If the dressing separates, then give it a vigorous shake before using or put the ingredients (i.e., olive oil and vinegar) on your food separately. It doesn't matter if it is separate or not.

Look carefully at the ingredients before you buy or eat an item. Emulsifiers have names such as these:

- citric acid esters
- polysorbates
- sorbitan tristearate

Thankfully most grocery stores and health-food stores have plenty of options today that are emulsifier free. Simply do a little homework before buying the foods you need, or go natural and make them at home.

IT'S A FACT

Emulsifiers cause inflammation in your gut—and your brain.[55]

You don't want emulsifiers mixing it up in your gut. The result is usually dysbiosis, leaky gut, and poor health.

COMMON ENEMY 7: SATURATED FATS

Another common enemy to your gut is saturated fat. The word *fat* might sound terrible, but the right types of fat, especially extra-virgin olive oil, avocado oil, and most nuts,[*] are both good for you and a necessary part of a healthy body.

Most saturated fat in our diets comes from meats or animal products, but plants also contain saturated fat. The primary sources of saturated fats include these:

- beef
- butter
- cheese
- cocoa butter
- coconut milk
- coconut oil
- cream
- ice cream
- pork
- sour cream
- palm oil

A simple test is to look at fats at room temperature. If fats are in a solid state at room temperature, then they are saturated fats and should be avoided or minimized. If they are liquid, such as avocado oil or olive oil, then they are unsaturated fats or monounsaturated fats and are better for consumption.

Within the unsaturated fat category is a subcategory known as polyunsaturated fats. I recommend avoiding or at least minimizing polyunsaturated fats, such as corn oil, soybean oil, and others, since many are GMO and they fuel inflammation.

_____

[*] Unless you are allergic to nuts

One challenge with avoiding saturated fats is that they are commonly found in processed foods, such as coffee creamers, baked desserts, non-dairy whips, products with cocoa, and more. You don't even know they are there. This is an important reason to avoid processed foods as much as possible.

When we have a high intake of saturated fat, we put our health at risk. A diet high in saturated fat has long been known to increase cholesterol levels, which may increase the risk of cardiovascular disease.[56]

There are also health risks that directly concern the gut. Saturated fat causes the release of lipopolysaccharide (LPS), an endotoxin that is bad for your gut and gut wall. LPS is naturally present in the outer membrane of gram-negative bacteria in your body. It helps protect the bacteria from being digested by bile acids.[57] When these bacteria die, the LPS is usually cleaned up and excreted by the liver.[58]

However, if the gut is already damaged with a leaky gut, the LPS pieces end up passing between the cells of the damaged gut wall and directly into your bloodstream. This causes inflammation in the body and can eventually trigger inflammation in your brain! LPS can increase beta-amyloid in the brain, which is a protein commonly found in the brains of Alzheimer's patients.[59]

Besides high-fat diets and an already leaking gut, other causes of LPS being released into your body include infections, overeating, drinking too much alcohol, dysbiosis (excessive amounts of bad bacteria), stress, and smoking.[60]

IT'S A FACT

LPS raises beta-amyloid protein levels. This protein is found at higher levels in people living with Alzheimer's and Parkinson's.[61]

Specifically, the LPS are adept at slipping through your gut wall and out into your body by "riding on and hiding in saturated fats."[62] That is how saturated fats play such an important role with LPS and your gut.

When LPS gets past your gut wall and into your bloodstream, inflammation is the direct result, and as you know, that can lead to a lot of sickerness, ailments, and autoimmune diseases. A few specific LPS-related symptoms include these:

- blood-clotting disorders
- fever
- leukocytosis (high white blood cell count)
- low iron levels
- platelet aggregation
- thrombocytopenia (low platelets)[63]

Studies have also found that LPS in your bloodstream can lead to obesity and type 2 diabetes.[64] And in men, LPS has been found to increase obesity and lower testosterone levels.[65]

Quite clearly, you do not want LPS floating around in your body. As expected, high LPS levels in the blood mean the gut is leaking, and you are usually consuming too many saturated fats. The healthier someone is, the lower his or her levels of LPS.

Alternatives/options/choices

Your doctor can test you for LPS with a blood test called the Cyrex Array 2 Intestinal Antigenic Permeability screen. The test looks for specific antibodies that are signs of LPS in the body, especially the LPS IgA and the LPS IgM antibody tests.

IT'S A FACT

Once the body mounts an immune defense, it is trained to react in the same way next time you eat the same food.

I perform this test with many of my sicker patients and consistently find that the sicker they are, the more ailments or symptoms they might have. They also typically have higher amounts of LPS floating around in their blood, and they usually consume too much saturated fat.

An added challenge with LPS is that it takes considerable time to lower these numbers. That is because the inflammation from LPS circulates through the entire body, and it takes time to clear up all that inflammation.

The Healthy Gut Zone diet, described in greater detail in chapter 11 of this book, works well to effectively lower LPS levels.

At a glance, here are three simple tools that help lower LPS levels:

1. Decrease saturated fat consumption significantly. This means coming off the typical keto-type diet with excessive amounts of saturated fats, such as butter, cream, cheese, coconut oil, and fatty meats. Medium-chain triglycerides and MCT oil from coconuts do not raise LPS levels, but coconut oil does.

2. Increase fish oil (omega 3) intake.

3. Consume a significant number of probiotics.

The Healthy Gut Zone diet will take you through more steps to lower your LPS, but even with only these three steps I've just mentioned, most patients experience excellent results.

Scientists have tested the effects of probiotics to lower LPS levels. In one study, in a mere four weeks, people saw a 42 percent drop in LPS levels and a 24 percent drop in triglyceride levels.[66]

That is a significant change from only probiotics. Add all the other strategies and parts of the Healthy Gut Zone diet, and you can rest assured that your LPS levels will go even lower and eventually to normal.

You must always remember that a leaky gut leads to food sensitivities and usually LPS circulating in your blood.[67] You do not want LPS in your body since it affects the gut and the body and will eventually trigger inflammation in the brain.

COMMON ENEMY 8: CONSTIPATION

What is one of the most common gut problems people have? Constipation. According to the Mayo Clinic, you are constipated if you experience fewer than three bowel movements per week.[68] This common enemy causes many problems, including these:

- pain and bleeding: hemorrhoids and anal tears (fissures), common results of straining too hard while trying to defecate

- bloating and discomfort: feeling nauseated, bloated, and gassy
- diverticulosis/diverticulitis: diverticula (abnormal pouches in the large intestinal lining, mainly on the left side and especially in the sigmoid colon) becoming infected and inflamed

Other effects of compacted stools are no fun to discuss, but some people end up in surgery to remove a segment of the colon, especially from recurrent diverticulitis.

Constipation is considered chronic when its symptoms last for at least three months.[69] An estimated 16 percent of people in the US suffer from chronic constipation,[70] and that leads to about 2.5 million doctor visits and more than 700,000 emergency room visits every year![71]

IT'S A FACT

Your gut needs movement. Food needs to move along in your gut, or excessive bad bacteria will grow.[72]

Here is something that most people have not considered: "The best parameter for assessing constipation is not *how often* you need to go to the toilet, but *how difficult* it is."[73] A person should have a bowel movement one to three times a day, and we are not talking about diarrhea. (In chapter 9 we will talk more about poop and what the different types mean, but for now, overcoming constipation is the goal.)

Just as travel often brings infections and diarrhea, it can also cause constipation. The disruption of what is normal, from foods to exercises to schedules to not sitting on your own toilet—all of it can easily cause constipation. All that to say, your gut is a real creature of habit.

Stress is another cause of constipation. It's almost as if the body focuses on the worry and shuts down everything else. That is pretty much what happens! Another cause of constipation is sluggish or low thyroid. This impairs gut movement, which brings constipation.

So much that affects your immune system, brain, mood, and overall health happens in your gut. Because of this, if there is constipation, the body is forced to work in slow motion. Your gut needs to be able to process foods in about twenty-four to forty-eight hours. Good gut motility (the muscles working properly) is a necessary part of your good health. In other words, constipation should not be a regular part of your daily routine. If it is, you need to do what it takes to restore your gut health.

Alternatives/options/choices

At first glance, there are many natural, inexpensive, and easy-to-implement ways to decrease constipation, improve gut motility, and be regular. Simple methods or ingredients include these:

- fiber (psyllium husk powder)
- water (drinking plenty every day)
- magnesium supplements (since people are often low)
- buffered vitamin C powder in water daily (starting low and going slow)

Fruit does, of course, have fiber, but fruit is also high in sugar, which is not the best thing for your gut health. Psyllium husk powder is fiber without any sugar, and it's inexpensive. (Refer to appendix D for recommended supplements.)

In addition, you can do the following:

- Take a brisk walk since exercise stimulates gut movement.
- Jump on a rebounder; it can be even better than walking.
- Drink hot tea, such as Smooth Move tea (which contains herbs that gently stimulate your intestines).
- Add probiotics to your diet.
- Take natural desiccated thyroid extract (a prescription) if your thyroid is low or sluggish.
- Drink a green phytonutrient-rich drink that contains organic grasses and foods rich in chlorophyll.
- Take magnesium citrate in liquid or capsule form (400–800 mg or more per day).

There is one more step that can help tremendously with constipation. It is this:

- Sit correctly on a toilet.

It is as simple as putting a small footstool (six to eight inches tall), such as a Squatty Potty, under your feet while seated on a toilet. The footstool lines up your intestines in more of a straight track, which decreases the amount of pressure needed to pass a stool. Think "runway" and "slingshot" at the same time, and the whole sitting and positioning thing will make sense.

Some poke fun at using a small footstool for this, but if you struggle with constipation, give it a try. It might be the missing piece that helps you the most.

If you are planning on traveling, here are a few additional steps you can take to help reduce the risk of constipation while you are away from your usual routine:

- Try to eat the foods you usually eat.
- Keep drinking lots of water.
- Take magnesium supplements with you.
- Continue to take fiber (psyllium husk powder) once or twice daily.
- Don't pressure yourself. Go when you need to.

Because your gut is a creature of habit, creating good habits will go a long way in your being regular. That is the goal, which is part of your overall plan for restoring the health of your gut. And when your gut is healthy, constipation will be a thing of the past!

COMMON ENEMY 9: STRESS

Stress has always been an enemy of the gut. Emotional, mental, and psychological strain, in addition to physical pain, are very real stresses, and your body pays the price for them.

Technically speaking, as it relates to your GI tract, stress increases your cortisol levels, and cortisol increases gut permeability (makes your gut more likely to leak) and usually causes inflammation throughout your body.[74] It creates a cycle of increased cortisol followed by gut leaking and inflammation, then more cortisol followed by more leaking and inflammation, with no end in sight.

IT'S A FACT

Chronic stress, even if it's "not all that bad," is harder on your body than intense, acute stress. Deal with stressors for the sake of good gut health.

Stress slows down digestion time, which helps the bad bacteria and harms the good. It also reduces the proper absorption of nutrients and minerals in the foods you eat. I have seen it mess with people's metabolisms, which caused them to gain weight.

Conversely, the stronger and healthier your gut is, the better you can handle stress. Dr. Perlmutter says, "I marvel at the thought that my gut's bugs, rather than my brain, can control my response to stress."[75]

When you have a healthy gut, stress makes less of a negative impact on your gut and your body. And when you finally subdue whatever the stresses are in your life, your gut health will automatically improve.

Alternatives/options/choices

Thankfully, you can usually reverse the negative effects of stress. It may take time and effort, but reversing the damage from stress is entirely possible.

The goal, of course, is to get free of whatever is stressing you. In many cases, patients are dealing with toxic emotions, unresolved emotional trauma, unforgiveness, or the pain of deceit, betrayal, rejection, anger—all of which negatively affect the gut.

When they resolve the issues and move on—when they forgive and release—the gut usually improves significantly. Holding on to unforgiveness and bitterness leads to gut issues every single time. I can't tell you how many patients I have had over the years who were holding onto their stressors. When they finally let go, their gut was able to heal.

Also, being too busy with too many obligations causes a lot of stress. Decrease your obligations, cut back your schedule, and get into God's rhythm. Busyness and being out of God's rhythm used to be my most significant source of stress.

Some stresses are more external than internal, meaning that you are in no way responsible for the pressure that is acting on you. Maybe a relationship, job, health issue, or other situation is a constant stress in your life, and there is nothing you can do to remove the stress. In that setting, I still encourage patients to work to get their gut as healthy as possible. That is often the best way to cope with stress.

Probiotics may help you cope with stress, especially these: *Bifidobacterium infantis, Lactobacillus helveticus, Bifidobacterium longum*, and *Bifidobacterium bifidum*. You can get supplements for these probiotics or find foods that provide you with these necessary stress-fighting bacteria. For example, natural sources of *Bifidobacterium infantis* include these:

- green olives
- kefir (goat or coconut)
- kimchi
- miso
- natto
- pickles
- sauerkraut
- tempeh
- yogurt (goat or coconut)[76]

Adaptogenic herbs such as ashwagandha, Panax ginseng, and rhodiola help many with stress issues. CBD oil capsules, L-theanine, Relora (magnolia bark extract), and dihydrohonokiol-B (DHH-B) are also beneficial for stress and are nonaddictive. One of my favorite supplements that helps most patients with stress and IBS is Cannab CBD oil from Designs for Health.

The bottom line with stress is twofold: remove the stressor if you can, but always work to strengthen your gut. A strong gut is your best defense.

COMMON ENEMY 10: STAYING TOO CLEAN

The last common enemy of the gut may seem a little outrageous, but it makes sense when you see the facts. This common enemy is staying too clean.

Cleanliness is said to be next to godliness, but it seems we have gotten a bit carried away with our efforts to eradicate bacteria in our homes, on our hands, and in the air. According to Dr. Giulia Enders:

> The higher the hygiene standards in a country, the higher that nation's incidence of allergies and autoimmune diseases. The more sterile a household is, the more its members will suffer from allergies and autoimmune diseases.[77]

It turns out that being too clean is not all that good for your body's bacteria. You know that a battle is always in place to keep the right balance of good and bad bacteria in your gut. The skin cleansers that you use may be helping the bad bacteria more than the good![78]

Some argue that you should go all natural and wash less, use less soap, skip using deodorants, and be okay with a little dirt. I encourage you to consider your daily routine and use wisdom. How far you take "going natural" is really up to you.

Being clean and reducing bacteria is fine, but trying to live in a sterile world (home, body, office) without dirt or bacteria takes things too far. Children need the exposure to dirt and microbes from parks, football fields, farms, etc. (not slums) to train their immune systems. Inadequate exposure to germs usually means that their immune systems are poorly equipped to deal with many health issues they will encounter. It's okay to get dirty. Kids need to run and play—and so do you. And your kids don't need a bath or shower every single night.

IT'S A FACT

"More than 95 percent of the world's bacteria are harmless to humans."[79]

Alternatives/options/choices

One way to reduce bacteria with washing, cleaning, or skin-care products is to buy or make natural skin cleansers so that you don't kill off the good bacteria. Another option is to use mild natural, organic cleansers such as pure-castile soap, but sparingly, mainly in the armpits and groin and not the rest of your body. Online, you will find countless recipes to meet your needs.

Again, it's up to your discretion as to how far you want to go. But staying too clean can hurt you more than it helps. Keep that in mind as you work to improve your gut health.

CHAPTER SEVEN

THE STEPS TO GUT DAMAGE

S ANDY LOST THIRTY-FIVE pounds by changing jobs. It had nothing to do with going on a diet or working to improve her gut health. She simply went from sitting behind a desk in an accounting office with twenty other middle-aged, overweight people to giving tours to groups of children at a local museum. Her environment changed, and that affected her weight, eating schedule, available foods, exercise routine, and much more.

The reverse usually happens as people often get sedentary jobs after college—driving to work, sitting down all day, going to happy hour after work, and then getting home late—and begin to gain weight.

Did their genes change? No, not at all. Were their genes always predisposed to a heavier weight? I would argue not, but some would say it's in the genes.

Regardless, if Sandy were to quit her museum job and go back to the desk, she would most likely gain back those thirty-five pounds. And if another health factor improved by switching jobs, she probably would see the reverse take place as well.

Again, it's not a gene issue. The environment plays a part, as do her genes. How much of your body is controlled by genes, and how much is controlled by choices, environment, and habits?

All of it plays a part, but I will say this: never let any excuse keep you from what you want. Any excuse is always just that—an excuse. Yes, genes or some other factor can play a part, but that is not the whole story. There is more to the equation.

FROM HEALTH TO SICKNESS

Years ago, I read about identical twin brothers who were incredibly different. One was a smoker, obese, and suffering from type 2 diabetes, while the other was a nonsmoker, lean, and healthy. They had the same genes, but everything else about them seemed to be opposites.

Nature versus nurture has been a long-standing debate, but I say all that to say this: you get to choose. That is always the case. Always keep this truth in mind, and use it as a source of encouragement and hope.

Now, with this understanding, here is the typical eight-step pattern for most people's decline in health.

Step 1: Genetics

Suppose you have three friends who are genetically predisposed to three health risks: obesity, high blood pressure, and arthritis. It's in their genes. They may even have parents or relatives who were sick or died from these or related diseases, but your three friends do not yet suffer from any of these genetic predispositions. It may be in their genes, but they are not aware of it.

Step 2: Triggers

Then something happens that triggers the genes of your three friends. Maybe it is something they eat, but most likely, it is something major that does significant damage to their guts. One of the seven causes of a leaky gut from chapter 4 would be sufficient. Maybe one friend travels and gets an intestinal infection, another takes several doses of antibiotics to fight a persistent urinary tract infection (UTI), and the third takes acid blockers to stop bothersome reflux.

To review, the seven causes of a leaky gut are antibiotics, NSAIDs, acid blockers, GMO foods, chlorine, pesticides, and intestinal infections. Whatever the cause for each of your friends, it is enough to activate those silent genes. Symptoms of obesity, high blood pressure, and arthritis may begin to appear.

Step 3: Environments

Your *environment* is defined as a consistent state of repeated exposure to whatever is around you. For example, if you work outside every day, fresh air is part of your environment. But your three friends are exposed to environments that chip away at and slowly undermine their good health. The ten common enemies we discussed in chapter 6 are gluten; a high-sugar, high-carb diet; dairy; lectins; artificial sweeteners; emulsifiers; saturated fats; constipation; stress; and staying too clean.

Maybe your three friends have a diet of gluten and nightshades (that was my damaging environment) or other foods full of sugar, artificial sweeteners, or saturated fats that leave their bodies open for sickness.

Step 4: Time

We are all creatures of habit, at least to some degree. We have favorite foods, drinks, clothes, smells, tastes, sports, books, music, movies, TV shows, or even driving routes. Once we find something we like, we tend to stick with it. We run into trouble when the behavior we are repeating is bad for our health. Doing it over and over is the perfect setup, hurting the bacteria balance in your gut, increasing gut permeability, and creating more inflammation and more symptoms, all of which slowly degrade your health. Over time, everything bad usually gets worse because of our habits.

Step 5: Leaky gut

At this point your three friends experience leaky gut, which is what happens to most people on their journeys to poor health. Bad bacteria, toxins, lectins, partially digested nutrients, and more begin to increasingly flow between the cells of the gut wall. Inflammation increases, and eventually, it breaks down the blood/brain barrier, setting the stage for inflammation in the brain.

Step 6: Inflammation

Inflammation is everywhere. Your three friends gain weight, have high blood pressure that keeps climbing, and experience joint aches and joint stiffness they've never had before. Inflammation affects everyone differently, and your three friends have individual genetic weaknesses that combine with the inflammation to make things even worse. Naturally, they turn to their doctors and get prescriptions to deal with their symptoms. Unfortunately, nothing improves.

Step 7: Autoimmunity

Because of the inflammation and the toxins or partially digested foods and inflammatory mediators passing into the bloodstream, the immune systems of your three friends get confused and begin to attack their tissues. There are no outside invaders, just internal miscommunication. This is how autoimmunity occurs: when a person's immune system attacks his or her own body and damages healthy cells, tissues, and organs as a result.

The brain is eventually affected, which may cause brain fog, poor memory, depressed or anxious mood, and problems focusing and concentrating.

Step 8: Disease

The cycle is now complete and will remain ongoing. If nothing is done to break free, your three friends will usually find themselves dealing with the following:

- arthritis (joint aches, swelling, stiffness, and eventually loss of function and autoimmune disease)
- high blood pressure (increased risk for heart attacks, atherosclerosis, and strokes)
- obesity (and more than twenty-five diseases directly associated with it[1])

Inflammation brings with it so many different conditions. Remember the old science law we learned in school, that an object in motion tends to stay in motion? Metaphorically, this is going to happen to your three friends unless they do something different.

These are the eight steps to gut damage, moving from health to sickness. Once you take these steps, you are at the door of disease. And unless you do something about it, that door will remain open!

CHAPTER EIGHT

NINE GUT DISEASES

SOME PEOPLE ARE willing to do whatever it takes to get healthy again. Others, though it seems illogical, refuse to quit eating or drinking the very things that caused their health problems in the first place. For example, I have had many patients with type 2 diabetes (especially males) who had a hard time giving up sweets (especially ice cream), but lowering blood sugar levels is vital for helping type 2 diabetic patients.

As you can imagine, the more serious the diagnosis, the more willing people are to give up their favorite things. Many years ago, I had a diabetic patient who was given a very serious diagnosis of diabetic ulcers on his feet and recurrent cellulitis. The doctor told him, "Change your eating habits, or you will probably lose one or both feet and possibly either leg."

He had motivation! He also had children and wanted to be part of their lives, running and playing with them outside. Being confined to a wheelchair would have ruined that opportunity.

Because what goes on in the gut is behind the scenes, patients are often slow to make necessary changes. They tend to wait until the symptoms accumulate and have progressed to a point where it is challenging for the body to heal itself.

My advice is always to trace the symptoms back to the root cause. Fix that real issue, and things typically start to clear up!

And here is some more good news about gut health: once your gut has been rebalanced and healed, you can usually enjoy your favorite foods or drinks, only in smaller quantities and less often than before. I can eat a little gluten and occasional peppers and tomatoes (nightshades that I know my body doesn't like), but only in small amounts. I can rotate them every three to four days and they cause no harm. That's better than none at all!

A healed gut usually reduces and removes most food sensitivities, but food allergies will generally remain. As for the diseases that come from long-term exposure to a leaky gut, most conditions improve once the gut has been healed.

IT'S A FACT

Make it a habit to eat more plants, raw or steamed. It feeds the good bacteria in your gut. And eat the whole thing, such as the broccoli or asparagus stem.

Every person is different, which simply means that every sickness plays out uniquely with each patient. Two people may have the same disease but different symptoms. I have seen that many times. But usually, when you address the core issue, the body heals itself. That is the amazing thing about the gut!

DISEASES IN THE GUT

Disease can occur at any point along the GI tract. Here are the nine most common diseases that typically start in the gut:

1. acid reflux/GERD
2. ulcers
3. IBS
4. ulcerative colitis
5. Crohn's disease
6. SIBO/SIFO
7. celiac disease
8. brain-related diseases
9. autoimmune diseases

If you have one of these or know someone who does, always remember that a healed gut potentially has the power to heal your entire body. No, it is not a guarantee, but I have seen so many bodies restored to good health *after fixing the gut* that I can confidently tell you: fix your gut, and the odds are in your favor that your symptoms, sickness, ailments, and disease will improve or may clear up entirely.

I have seen the impossible happen so many times that I take a new patient's grim diagnosis with a grain of salt. "I really don't think it's as bad as you've been told" is not what doctors usually say, but it is true. And patients breathe a sigh of relief when they hear it.

So, whatever you are facing, no matter how discouraging or depressing it might be, let me say this: I don't think it's as bad as you've been told. The first step is to get your gut healthy again.

GUT DISEASE 1: ACID REFLUX/GERD

The most common disease of the gut, the disease that generates the most doctor visits about the gut, is acid reflux or gastroesophageal reflux disease (GERD). It is estimated that more than sixty million people in the US have acid reflux at least once per month.[1] I would guess that more than 50 percent of my patients have this.

With acid reflux or GERD, a person's stomach acid seeps backward up the GI tract and damages the mucus lining of the esophagus. Here are a few of the most common symptoms:

- excessive saliva: production of a lot of saliva, similar to when one is about to vomit
- heartburn: hot burning sensation in the chest, just above the stomach
- nausea: varies from a stomachache to vomiting
- regurgitation: acidic burps
- sore throat: pain and trouble swallowing after meals[2]

What is the typical response when people have these symptoms? Naturally, they run to a grocery store to buy antacids or other acid-blocking medications or to their doctor to request something more substantial.

IT'S A FACT

The cause of acid reflux is often obesity, not the presence of too much stomach acid.[3]

For "something stronger," doctors regularly prescribe proton pump inhibitors (PPIs) that turn off your stomach acid and reduce acid secretion by 66–80 percent.[4] These PPIs do the job and then some! But studies are finding that PPIs may also increase your risk of cardiovascular disease, chronic kidney disease, dementia, pneumonia, gastric cancer, *Clostridium difficile* infections, and more.[5]

As always, treating the symptoms will usually not fix the core issue. Removing or lowering stomach acid is not going to fix anything long term. The truth is, it only makes matters worse.

The problem

Did you know that the mere act of swallowing uses thirty different nerves and muscles in unison? The muscles you control and feel (called striated muscles) are the ones in your tongue and throat. Once you swallow, the muscles you cannot directly control (called smooth muscles) automatically take over, pushing whatever you swallowed down your esophagus and into your stomach.[6]

Cranial nerves, as well as nerves in the mouth and the esophagus, control these muscles.[7] As we age, we lose some of the natural ability for our muscles (both the smooth and striated muscles) to work in perfect harmony. That is partly why the younger population seldom has acid reflux issues.

Another age-related fact is that our acid levels decline as we age. I find this interesting, because people usually take more antacids or acid blockers as they age.

The whole issue with acid reflux and acid being allowed back up the GI tract, out of the stomach and into the esophagus area, is most often due to nerves in your smooth muscles failing to work properly. Specifically, one sphincter muscle or valve between the esophagus and stomach, called the lower esophageal sphincter (LES), at times pops open, allowing for the brief backward movement of stomach acid. That means acid reflux is usually a valve or muscle issue and not a stomach acid issue at all!

When it comes to acid reflux and GERD, the millions of prescriptions written and billions of dollars spent on antacid and acid-blocking medications every year are an exercise in futility!

The problem made worse

To make matters worse is the fact that antacids and acid-blocking meds mess up your gut by killing good bacteria, which are in place not only to help digest your food and absorb nutrients but also to protect your body from allergens, bacteria, and toxins.[8]

Whether we have less stomach acid because we are getting older or because we are taking antacids or acid-blocking medications, the result is the same: an increased risk for these conditions:

- accelerated aging
- allergies
- bacterial overgrowth in the stomach and small intestine
- depression
- gall bladder disease
- Graves' disease
- lupus
- osteoporosis
- pernicious anemia
- poor absorption of essential vitamins, minerals, and amino acids
- poor digestion of proteins
- rheumatoid arthritis
- skin disease (acne, dermatitis, eczema, and hives)
- stomach cancer
- type 1 diabetes[9]

We need our stomach acid! One of the primary reasons these diseases have a chance in the first place is because we have removed our body's natural first line of defense—our stomach acid.

IT'S A FACT

The common reasons the sphincter muscle/valve between the stomach and esophagus dilates, causing acid reflux, include these:

- » *age (muscles not working in unison)[10]*
- » *being overweight or obese (causes pressure)[11]*
- » *consuming too much at dinner[12]*
- » *drinking coffee, alcohol, and milk[13]*
- » *eating chocolate, peppermint, garlic, onions, and citrus[14]*
- » *eating fatty foods[15]*
- » *eating spicy foods, including tomatoes and peppers[16]*
- » *eating too quickly[17]*
- » *food allergies and food sensitivities[18]*
- » *gravity (lying flat in bed)[19]*
- » *medications, including Viagra, Cialis, NSAIDs, and heart meds[20]*
- » *smoking[21]*
- » *stress[22]*
- » *wearing shapewear[23]*

Without stomach acid to properly break down and absorb proteins, vitamins, calcium, and other nutrients, it is a pretty direct route to low bone density and eventually bone fractures.[24]

When calcium, for example, can't get into the bloodstream through the gut wall because no stomach acid is there to do the conversion and absorption, then it is impossible for the much-needed calcium to reach the bones![25] I have seen many other debilitating issues, such as sarcopenia (frailty syndrome) and arthritis, come as a direct result of this. The sad news is that these deficiency-related ailments are preventable!

You already know that stomach acid kills bad bacteria. So taking acid-blocking meds allows bad bacteria to multiply, outnumbering the good, and leads to bacteria overgrowth. Ironically the symptoms of bad bacteria overgrowth in the small intestines—such as gas, bloating, and belching—mimic acid reflux.[26] And taking more acid blockers is what most people do in response!

An additional irony is that heartburn, often called the telltale sign of acid reflux, is usually a signal that the stomach has too little stomach acid, not too much.[27] Again, the main issue is the sphincter muscle, not the acid in the stomach that seeps back up into the esophagus.

IT'S A FACT

One study found that more than 30 percent of people over age sixty suffer from atrophic gastritis, where they have very little or no stomach acid at all.[28]

Acid blockers are not just for adults. We are even using them on babies. Doctors regularly prescribe antacids to babies who spit up after feeding. Instead, I suggest frequent small feedings and sitting the baby in a reclining seat or a car seat at a forty-five-degree angle or higher for thirty to sixty minutes after feedings to prevent reflux. But no acid-blocking prescriptions! That will not be good for the baby's GI tract, either now or in the future.

Here is another sad example of the many issues that arise when we blindly try to stamp out stomach acid, and I have seen it countless times:

A man with erectile dysfunction (ED) issues often takes Viagra, which regularly results in acid reflux. He then gets medication to stop the stomach acid, which then usually leads to SIBO or IBS. After a round of antibiotics, leaky gut starts, followed by inflammation and brain fog. Eventually autoimmune disease may develop, as well as leaky brain with memory problems, weight gain, and more.

It is quite a train of sickness, and it all started over ED issues, which may have resulted from low testosterone levels and circulation issues brought on from his being obese.

Here is another technical point: Most people cannot have too much stomach acid. It doesn't work that way. With the exception of a few rare medical conditions, our bodies will not produce too much acid. They create just enough. The point is, you need your stomach acid!

Alternatives/options/choices

Why do antacids work? Because they lower acid levels and give the malfunctioning LES muscle a break. But turning off stomach acid for months and then years at a time is not good for your gut health![29]

As much as you need your stomach acid, having acid reflux is no fun. While you are working to restore your gut's health, here are a few tips to immediately reduce acid reflux:

- Drink alkaline water.
- Sip hot tea or water regularly.
- Lay off peppermints, caffeine, chocolate, and alcohol.
- Avoid foods that make you bloat.
- Eat smaller meals, especially at dinner.
- Take smaller bites and chew each bite well.
- Chew gum, which keeps saliva running downhill.
- Elevate the head of your bed by thirty degrees.
- Try deglycyrrhizinated licorice (DGL) with mastic gum (order online).
- Lose weight, especially belly fat.
- Avoid tight belts, shapewear, or girdles.
- Take Endefen, which contains plantain and apple pectin along with cinnamon and a few other natural ingredients that relieve reflux (order online).
- Add ginger to foods or water.
- Take aloe vera.

- Take one to two digestive enzymes at the beginning of your meal.

- Try apple cider vinegar. One teaspoon to 1 tablespoon in a glass of water before or after meals may reduce reflux symptoms.

The best long-term answer to acid reflux is to get your gut healthy again. That will include your sphincter muscle at the top of your stomach. A healthy gut will usually give your sphincter muscle the break it needs and enough time to heal itself. Though it is a muscle, it's not like you can lift weights to strengthen it. Rest, relaxation, weight loss, and eating smaller meals are significant factors in getting it strong again.

IT'S A FACT

As we age, our digestive enzymes become depleted and it becomes necessary to take a digestive enzyme supplement.

Follow the Healthy Gut Zone diet, decrease stress, and remove medications and foods that relax your LES. You will find that your sphincter muscle will almost always be back in shape in a few months.

GUT DISEASE 2: ULCERS

Another common gut disease is ulcers. Ulcers are open sores in the GI tract from mouth to anus, but usually located in the stomach and small intestines, that may fester, ooze pus, bleed, and create holes at any point along the way.

Every year, almost 6 percent (14.8 million) of adults in the US are diagnosed with ulcers.[30] Usually, it is the older population that suffers from ulcers, but many teens and even preteens are being diagnosed these days as well.

Ulcers have different names depending on where they are located in your GI tract and what they are doing (i.e., bleeding or not), but they all are about the same. When the protective mucus coating of the GI tract is weakened, stomach acid and bad bacteria break through to the sensitive lining below, and that causes irritation, pain, and the ulcer.[31]

The typical symptoms of ulcers that patients bring into my offices include the following:

- blood in the stool (or in vomit)
- eating actually hurts
- lack of appetite
- nausea
- pain often described as burning in the stomach area
- vomiting
- weight loss

Ulcers are no fun at all!

Causes of ulcers

Despite what we have heard for years and years, stress, spicy foods, coffee, and too much stomach acid do not cause ulcers. Instead, bad bacteria—specifically, *H. pylori* bacteria—and nonsteroidal anti-inflammatory drugs (NSAIDs, such as ibuprofen and Naprosyn) cause ulcers.[32] In addition to ulcers, *H. pylori* is responsible for causing atrophic gastritis, where the body quits making stomach acid completely, and stomach cancer.[33]

H. pylori is bad news for your body, especially your gut. Look at it this way: "*H. pylori* can manipulate our protective barriers, irritate and destroy our cells, and manufacture toxins and damage our entire body by doing so."[34]

IT'S A FACT

*Stress, coffee, and select foods or drinks may aggravate existing ulcers, but they do **not** cause ulcers.*

Prescribed antacids or other acid-blocking medications make things worse because "reducing stomach acid makes life significantly easier for *H. pylori*" and increases inflammation and infection.[35] Because *H. pylori* is a type of bacteria, it can spread through contact with contaminated people, food, or water.[36]

Back in 1984, in front of a group of fellow doctors, Dr. Barry Marshall from Australia drank a petri dish of the *H. pylori* bacteria, and within days he was sick with gastritis, which is the precursor of ulcers. He effectively proved once and for all that ulcers were not caused by stress! It took ten more years for the medical community to acknowledge his breakthrough and twenty years for him to win a Nobel Prize for his efforts.

Ulcers in the GI tract leave physical evidence (cuts, holes, inflammation, blood, etc.), which means they can be detected with an X-ray or by endoscopy. But because ulcers are primarily driven by *H. pylori*, these bacteria can usually be found by using stool tests or breath tests and by taking a tissue sample from an endoscopy. The stool and breath tests are better at detecting active *H. pylori* infections than a blood test.[37]

When scientists discovered that *H. pylori* bacteria cause ulcers, everything changed for the better for those who suffer from ulcers and gastritis. It has become standard practice to check for this kind of bacteria, and that makes it so much easier.

Alternatives/options/choices

The usual treatment regimen for ulcers is a prescription of antibiotics for about two weeks and acid-blocking meds for two weeks. The antibiotics kill the harmful *H. pylori* (and a lot of other good bacteria), and the acid blocker is to calm the gut (less stomach acid burning in the ulcer spots on the stomach or GI tract wall) so that it has time to heal.[38]

IT'S A FACT

Mastic trees have natural ingredients (in capsules, powder, oil, toothpaste, and mouthwash) that help eliminate the **H. pylori** *bacteria.*[39]

Because the *H. pylori* bacteria destroy stomach acid, taking additional antacids can make things even worse. The bad bacteria have free rein when there is less stomach acid, which increases the risks for gastritis, ulcers, and stomach cancer.[40]

Although certain antibiotics do heal ulcers, we have also learned that antibiotics kill good bacteria in your gut. So, now that we know the cause of most ulcers is the bad *H. pylori* bacteria, is it possible to get rid of ulcers without antibiotics?

The answer is to use probiotics, such as *S. boulardii* and *Lactobacillus gasseri*, with antibiotics. This approach effectively kills off the bad *H. pylori* bacteria and gets the body back on track. One study found that giving patients *Lactobacillus gasseri*–containing yogurt with their antibiotics led to a higher rate (82.6 percent) of successfully eradicating *H. pylori*, compared to patients who received antibiotics alone (69 percent eradication rate).[41]

With ulcers, I recommend DGL and mastic gum to help calm the GI tract. I also recommend a specific antibiotic treatment for two weeks and include probiotics in the process. Then afterward, I instruct patients to pour on the probiotics to reverse the effects of antibiotics on the good gut bacteria.

GUT DISEASE 3: IBS

Another prevalent disease of the gut is IBS, or irritable bowel syndrome. Technically speaking, IBS is a functional disorder, meaning that your GI organs are normal but there are symptoms that something is wrong. In other words, most diagnostic tests "are designed to identify structural problems, but not disorders of function" such as IBS.[42] Not a good outlook on life!

As you know, with acid reflux, the lower esophageal sphincter between the stomach and esophagus fails to function correctly and lets stomach acid back up into the unprotected esophagus. But with IBS, it's different. In some IBS cases, another sphincter, the ileocecal valve between the large intestine and the small intestine, can be damaged. I have found that this can result from chronic irritation, inflammation, appendicitis, Crohn's disease, surgery for appendicitis, and other things that cause scar tissue in the sphincter muscle. This effectively leaves an opening for bad bacteria to migrate from the large intestine back up into the small intestine, and that brings with it all the irritating IBS symptoms! The small intestine does not usually have much bacteria in it, but when the sphincter valve is damaged and open, the backflow continues unchecked.

IBS is such a broad name that many sicknesses and diseases often start as an IBS diagnosis before they are further clarified. To increase the confusion, certain foods, stress, gluten, food allergies or sensitivities, and diseases can contribute to or cause IBS. Some get IBS after they have had a stomach or intestinal bacterial infection.[43] I have seen patients develop IBS after they had a leaky gut, candida, SIFO, or dysbiosis.

Here are a few of the most common symptoms of IBS:

- bloating and gas after eating
- constipation, diarrhea, or both
- duration of symptoms lasting from weeks to years
- feeling of not completely emptying after having a bowel movement
- intolerance to gluten, dairy (lactose), or fruits (fructose)
- lower abdominal pain, usually relieved after a bowel movement
- passage of mucus with a bowel movement

As you can see, these symptoms are pretty generic in regard to the gut. Food sensitivities and allergies have many of these same symptoms, as does celiac disease.

IBS is a name that often appears when dealing with the gut. I would estimate that about 25 percent of my patients have IBS. Approximately 10–15 percent of the US adult population suffers from IBS symptoms, yet only 5–7 percent have been diagnosed with the disease.[44]

IT'S A FACT

Most people with IBS learn to cope with it. But coping is not living!

The usual prescription that doctors give for IBS is an antispasmodic or antidepressant type of drug. That might be in part due to the fact the gut and brain are directly connected, and IBS sufferers say they can literally feel the pain in their gut. We now know that patients with IBS have an increased sensitivity to pain in the GI tract, and we call this visceral hypersensitivity. Visceral hypersensitivity, in turn, causes many with

IBS to misinterpret normal sensations in their GI tract as abnormal and painful.[45] But in any case, as you well know, an antispasmodic or antidepressant drug is not going to fix the core problems in the gut that cause IBS.

Gut bacteria in the mix

I had IBS many years ago, and as I mentioned earlier in this book, when I contracted the parasite giardia by water-skiing (and drinking the water) in a freshwater Florida lake, my IBS symptoms only got worse. Long after the giardia bacteria was gone, my IBS symptoms stuck around. In fact, I battled IBS for years. It did a number on my gut.

My experience with patients leads me to believe that IBS is mostly the result of a bacterial imbalance. Whatever the cause, the good bacteria in the gut are usually killed off, giving the bad bacteria free rein to grow, overpopulate, and mess with the entire GI tract.

Though the symptoms are obvious enough, there is no IBS test that doctors can administer. The lack of a specific test may prolong the sickness, but I have found that IBS usually clears up when the good gut bacteria gain the majority. Many patients with IBS turn out to have SIBO or SIFO (more on these later).

The Healthy Gut Zone diet, explained in greater detail in chapter 11, has repeatedly proven effective with hundreds of patients in overcoming their IBS.

Road map to avoiding IBS

Although IBS is pretty generic, hard to test for, and a challenge to overcome, we have known for years how to avoid IBS.

IT'S A FACT

IBS sufferers live an avoidance life. That is because they may have any or all of these:

» *lactose intolerance—and should avoid or minimize all dairy containing lactose, such as milk, yogurt, cheese, and ice cream*

» *fructose intolerance—and should avoid or minimize fruits, juices, berries, some vegetables (onions, artichokes, peas), and processed foods with fructose as a sweetener*

» *gluten sensitivity—and should avoid gluten found in wheat, barley, and rye*

» *fiber sensitivity—and should avoid or minimize fruits, veggies (broccoli, cauliflower, cabbage), legumes (beans, peas, lentils), and many, if not most, fiber supplements (Psyllium husk powder can be added later, but start with a low dose and go slow.)*

» *sorbitol sensitivity—and should avoid this sugar substitute commonly found in sugar-free candy, gums, etc.*[46]

A very specific diet eliminates foods that cause gas and bloating—specifically, any fermentable food. The idea is that if you remove the food that ferments, you also usually get rid of gas and bloating.

This is called the FODMAP (fermentable oligosaccharides, disaccharides, monosaccharides, and polyols) diet. It divides foods into two groups: those that are highly fermentable (which you should not eat) and those that are less fermentable (which you should eat). In his book *Take Control of Your IBS*, gastroenterologist Peter Whorwell gives these examples:[47]

FODMAP Categories

High in FODMAPs (Do not eat these)	Low in FODMAPs (Eat these)
apple	all fish
artificial sweeteners	all meat
blackberry	banana
bread (gluten)	blueberry
cauliflower	carrot

High in FODMAPs (Do not eat these)	Low in FODMAPs (Eat these)
cow's milk	egg
garlic and leeks	gluten-free bread
honey	lemon
mushroom	mandarin
onion	parsnip
peach	potato
pear	rhubarb
plum	rice
prune	sugar
sweet corn	swede
watermelon	turnip
	water

The FODMAP diet can help reduce gas and bloating, but again, it does not fix the real issues. Avoiding something is not an answer. It may help temporarily with symptoms, and it may even be advisable for the short-term, but getting rid of IBS requires fixing the gut and balancing the gut bacteria.

Alternatives/options/choices

IBS, with its general blanket of symptoms mixed with very real and painful food sensitivities, is completely curable. I see it happen all the time.

IT'S A FACT

Sensitive to gluten? It may be IBS and not celiac disease.[48]

Most people with IBS simply try to learn to live with it. Their valiant efforts are why IBS is called a functional disorder. The good news is that you don't have to live this way. You can be free of IBS.

In my practice, we treat the core issue behind IBS. We work to build the good bacteria back up to the proper level. That requires changing one's eating habits, reducing and then stopping medicines that are over-populating the bad bacteria, and adding specific supplements.

When you reduce the bad bacteria, you essentially remove the "engine" that causes the fermenting. A healthy gut does not have all the gas and bloating issues that people with IBS have to deal with, yet they could be eating the same foods.

It is usually an issue of excessive bad bacteria, inflammation of the gut (leaky gut), and certain foods that aggravate IBS. Also, we sometimes have to close the ileocecal valve that connects the small intestine to the large intestine. When it is open, bacteria come up from the colon and into the small intestine. In most cases, a combination of the Healthy Gut Zone diet and probiotics helps to restore normal bowel function. Fixing the bacterial balance and the gut is the surest way of fixing IBS. The process is not all that complicated and usually takes only a few months.

GUT DISEASE 4: SIBO/SIFO

The next common diseases of the gut are SIBO and SIFO, and their prevalence is increasing rapidly. Here is how they are defined:

- Small intestinal bacterial overgrowth (SIBO) "occurs when there is an abnormal increase in the overall bacterial population in the small intestine."[49]
- Small intestinal fungal overgrowth (SIFO) occurs when there is an "excessive number of fungal organisms in the small intestine associated with gastrointestinal (GI) symptoms."[50]

It is estimated that 10 percent of the entire global population has IBS (irritable bowel syndrome); of that number (seven hundred million), an estimated 60 percent also have SIBO.[51] Since between twenty-five and forty-five million Americans suffer from IBS,[52] that means about fifteen to twenty-seven million of those have SIBO! In addition, approximately 25 percent of patients with unexplained GI symptoms have SIFO.[53] That is a lot of pain and discomfort for a lot of people.

To make matters slightly worse, a lot of people diagnosed with IBS were aware of their symptoms for many years before they decided it was time to seek treatment.[54] That shows just how often IBS (and therefore SIBO and SIFO) are put up with, worked around, lived with, or accepted as normal.

IT'S A FACT

*The good bacteria in the gut directly impact your mood
by controlling your serotonin and dopamine levels.[55]*

Why are so many people suffering from SIBO and SIFO these days? The answer is gut damage from many outside sources (discussed in chapter 4), all of which contribute to or cause leaky gut. Add the usual foods and other enemies of the gut (discussed in chapter 6) that cause so much pain and damage after the gut has started to leak, and it only makes sense. And if this goes on for years and years, no wonder we have skyrocketing numbers of SIBO and SIFO cases.

I'll remind you of the stomach acid example. Your body needs stomach acid, and if you take antacids or more potent acid blockers to suppress stomach acid, you naturally end up with a low-acid to no-acid stomach. That results in bacteria and fungus having free rein to grow, multiply, and spread throughout your GI tract.[56] That is many times the cause of your SIBO and SIFO right there!

People are regularly diagnosed with dysbiosis, which is an excessive amount of bad bacteria in the gut. That is SIBO—when the excessive bacteria are in the small intestines where they do not belong.

SIFO, on the other hand, is a less common diagnosis. For many years, I would diagnose the symptoms of SIFO as candida because 97 percent of the time, a candida yeast or fungus is responsible for SIFO.[57] Candida is the overgrowth of yeast, often in the small intestine, which is exactly what SIFO is. I wrote *The Bible Cure for Candida and Yeast Infections* in 2001, but today that disease would be called SIFO.

Keep in mind that your body naturally has many different fungi in your gut, and candida is just one of them. The presence of candida in your small intestine may be typical, but the overgrowth is not.[58]

Symptoms of SIBO/SIFO

Many people with SIBO also have SIFO, and they share many common symptoms. Before we look at their symptoms, let's take a quick look at the symptoms of IBS. According to the Mayo Clinic and other medical personnel, IBS symptoms vary from patient to patient but can include the following:

- abdominal pain
- bloating
- brain fog
- constipation
- cramping
- diarrhea
- dizziness
- excessive gas
- fatigue
- mucus in the stool
- ringing in the ears[59]

This IBS list is admittedly very general, but so are many of the symptoms of SIBO and SIFO. Symptoms of SIBO and SIFO include these:

- abdominal pain
- belching
- bloating
- brain fog
- constipation
- cramping
- cravings for carbs and sugar
- depression
- diarrhea
- fatigue
- food sensitivities
- gas
- headaches

- impaired concentration
- irritability
- nail infections
- nausea
- oral thrush
- poor memory
- rashes
- rectal itching (SIFO)
- skin problems
- vaginal itching (SIFO)

When bad bacteria or fungi overpopulate your small intestines, your body pays the price, no matter what. These symptoms are a reflection of that reality.

With these general gut-related symptoms, however, it is understandable why doctors may diagnose someone with IBS but might not spend the time or even know how to diagnose (much less treat effectively) someone with SIBO or SIFO.

One leading cause of SIBO and SIFO is multiple rounds of broad-spectrum antibiotics.[60] As we mentioned earlier in this chapter, suppression of stomach acid is another cause behind IBS and therefore behind SIBO and SIFO. Risk factors for SIBO and SIFO include low stomach acid, constipation, diabetes, IBS, celiac disease, Crohn's disease, and bowel or abdominal surgery.[61]

In addition to antibiotic overuse and low stomach acid , other causes of SIBO and SIFO include these:

- blockage in the intestines[62]
- changes in the immune function of the GI tract[63]
- chronic constipation[64]
- diabetes[65]
- diverticula (abnormal pouches) in the gut wall[66]
- genetic predisposition[67]
- infection in the GI tract[68]

- inflammatory bowel disease (IBD)[69]
- neurological issues[70]
- surgery to the small or large intestine[71]
- various medications[72]

One seemingly small cause of SIBO and SIFO is constipation, but as we have previously discussed, it is a big problem with many damaging repercussions. With over fifty-two million (16 percent) of people in the US suffering from chronic constipation,[73] it is the perfect setup for SIBO and SIFO.

IT'S A FACT

If you bloat with a teaspoon of psyllium husk powder, you may have SIBO or SIFO. You still need the fiber, so start low and go slow. Start with one-quarter teaspoon a day, and you may be able (if you have no bloating or gas) to slowly work your way up to a full teaspoon one to two times a day (after breakfast and after dinner).

You see, the small intestine is responsible for 90 percent of all the calories absorbed from the food you eat and is home to most of your immune system cells.[74] For the small intestine to work efficiently, the food needs to pass through quickly (but not too quickly or diarrhea will occur), or bad bacteria and fungi will grow more rapidly. Constipation slows everything down.

When SIBO or SIFO is mixed with constipation, the bacteria or fungi have even more time to overpopulate in the small intestine. No wonder the symptoms of SIBO and SIFO are so unpleasant and usually missed by most physicians.

Testing for SIBO is typically done in two ways:

1. a breath test that measures excessive hydrogen and methane gas levels

2. a small bowel aspirate or a probe sent down to culture the contents in the small intestine

You cannot do a breath test for SIFO because an overgrowth of fungus does not release gas (from the fermenting process) like an overgrowth of bacteria does. In other words, fungal levels cannot be tested with a breath test, but bacterial levels can be.[75]

Because it is harder to test for SIFO, the disease is harder to diagnose. It is possible (as with SIBO testing) to have an endoscopy or a small bowel aspirate and take a culture sample from the small intestines to test for fungus (or bacteria), but these tests can be invasive and expensive. They also take time to prepare and administer.

IT'S A FACT

If you have IBS but do not have SIBO, then you probably have SIFO.

With my patients, I may do a SIBO breath test, but other than that, further testing will often prove only what we already know. They are suffering from gut issues, their symptoms are genuine, and by restoring the gut to a healthy state, the symptoms will almost always go away, provided we kill the excess fungus and bacteria.

IT'S A FACT

Gas usually forms in the colon (large intestine), and almost everything you eat and drink (except water) creates gas. That is part of the normal digestion and fermentation process in the GI tract. The most common gases in your gut are nitrogen, oxygen, hydrogen, carbon dioxide, and methane. Most gas (oxygen) comes from swallowing air while you are eating. Stinky gas (methane) is from fermenting foods in your colon.[76] Eating fewer carbs, sugars, and starches will result in less methane gas.

By treating the entire GI tract as an organ, I have found that patients not only understand the importance of gut health but are also more willing to do what it takes to get their gut functioning optimally again.

Alternatives/options/choices

As with any gut disease, the best remedy is always to restore your gut to good health. The Healthy Gut Zone diet in chapter 11 is where I immediately take patients who suffer from IBS, whether they know they have SIBO or SIFO yet or not. It works exceptionally well.

Because SIBO and SIFO are based on the improper balance of bacteria and fungi in the gut, rebalancing these two is the natural and most important step. I have found the most significant impact on bacteria and fungi comes through doing the following:

1. **Take probiotics.** Adding probiotics to the diet is especially effective. Probiotics have been found to kill off bad bacteria, so as with antibiotics, they help clear infections.[77] Most importantly for SIBO patients, they help correct dysbiosis. Use caution with prebiotics and fiber because they can make SIBO worse.[78] *Saccharomyces boulardii* is a yeast-based probiotic that may help both SIBO and SIFO.

2. **Starve the bad bacteria and bad fungi.** That simply means steering clear of bread, starches, and sugars. This is especially effective for SIFO patients.

3. **Kill excess bad bacteria and fungi.**

4. **Heal the leaky gut.**

Additional supplements and herbs are also helpful, but without taking these first steps, the rest will have a minimal impact. Herbs are especially effective in treating SIBO and SIFO because they help thin out the bad bacteria, yeast, and fungi, whether you have SIBO or SIFO. They are also inexpensive and readily available in most health-food stores.

For at least six weeks, I use these herbs to help my patients who are fighting SIBO or SIFO:

- Caprylic acid is usually effective against candida (yeast).
- berberine: active against candida and bacteria
- grapefruit seed extract: antibacterial and antifungal activity
- oil of oregano: active against fungus and bacteria

- Silver Biotics (not colloidal silver): antibacterial and antifungal activity; active against yeast and fungi

Need more beneficial health aspects of herbs? Their benefits include being antidepressant (oil of oregano), lowering and controlling blood sugar levels (berberine), and helping to reduce IBD symptoms (artemisinin). Artemisinin is also very good for many parasitic infections of the GI tract.

IT'S A FACT

People with chronic diarrhea often have SIBO or SIFO.

Fiber and prebiotics can sometimes make SIBO and SIFO worse. But when the bloating and gas have improved, I then add small amounts of psyllium husk powder, one-quarter to one-half teaspoon one or two times a day, gradually increasing the dose. If bloating and gas occur, decrease or stop fiber intake. Speeding up the flow of things through the intestines usually removes the perfect feeding ground for bad bacteria and fungus.

GUT DISEASE 5: CELIAC DISEASE

Another common gut disease is celiac disease. It is known around the world. Unfortunately, it can cause incredible pain and discomfort and even death. Celiac disease is defined as an autoimmune disease where the body overreacts to the smallest amount of gluten protein and damages the gut wall.

Approximately 1 percent or over three million people in the US have celiac disease. What is hard to imagine is that about 83 percent of people with celiac disease are undiagnosed or misdiagnosed for many years,[79] and this in itself leads to other sicknesses and diseases. According to different doctors from around the globe, the number of people thought to be gluten sensitive (not celiac) ranges from as low as 6 percent to as high as 50 percent![80] I think the gluten sensitivity that is so prevalent today is simply a reflection of all the gut issues discussed so far in this book. A leaky gut will naturally usually be sensitive to gluten, and without repairing the gut, the situation usually will get progressively worse.

In celiac disease, gluten sets off an autoimmune reaction that can eventually lead to the destruction of the villi that line the small intestines. This leads to malabsorption, usually weight loss, and chronic illness. Celiac disease affects one in 133 people in the US and "is twice as common as Crohn's disease, ulcerative colitis, and cystic fibrosis combined."[81]

Remember these two illustrations from earlier (in chapter 4)? They show the gut wall and how it is made of cells that have little villi (tiny fingerlike projections) on the inside (the side that touches the food you eat) and blood vessels on the other side that feed directly into your bloodstream. In a healthy gut, the villi help absorb the amino acids, fatty acids, sugars, and nutrients from what you eat.

In a gut where the little villi have been knocked off, flattened down, and destroyed, you end up with malabsorption of nutrients, a weakened immune system, inflammation, loss of bone density, leaky gut, miscarriages, infertility, and imminent sickness and disease.[82]

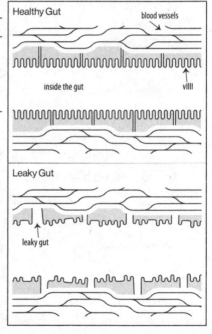

The damage to celiac patients' villi is much worse than in those who suffer from severe leaky gut syndrome. That is, if we compare the intestines of a celiac disease patient with those of someone who has damage from another cause of leaky gut (described in chapter 4), they may look similar, but the celiac patient's gut is much worse and usually has completely flattened villi.

Celiac patients need to strictly avoid all gluten. Currently there are no drugs to treat celiac disease, and there is no cure, so the only option is avoiding all products containing gluten, which includes wheat, barley, and rye and any product containing these grains.

Symptoms of celiac disease

People who have celiac disease usually know they must avoid gluten. Should they eat foods with gluten (see appendix C for a list of such foods), these common symptoms are sure to flare up:

- abdominal pain
- anemia
- bloating
- bone/joint pain
- constipation
- diarrhea
- fatigue
- gas
- heartburn
- headaches
- loss of bone density
- nausea
- nervous system injury (including numb or tingling hands or feet, balance problems, or changes in awareness)
- rash (itchy, blistery)
- reduced spleen function
- ulcers in the mouth
- weight loss[83]

Celiac has long been considered hereditary, but with the increasing rates of celiac disease, people are wondering if other factors (such as the overuse of antibiotics,[84] NSAIDs, acid blockers, etc.) could be causes.

IT'S A FACT

Children with celiac disease are at a higher risk for type 1 diabetes.[85]

Nobody wants celiac disease, and it is not contagious. Still, anyone can end up with a damaged gut and similar symptoms of celiac disease if one allows his or her GI tract health to deteriorate. And because almost all autoimmune diseases share the common denominator of having a leaky gut, the goal must be that of restoring your gut to a healthy condition.

Alternatives/options/choices

If you have celiac disease, you simply must avoid gluten. This limitation is forever. You can live a fully functioning life by going gluten-free.

Restoring your gut health will naturally help decrease other related symptoms, sicknesses, and diseases. But you will need to stay off gluten. If you have damaged your gut to the point that it functions similarly to someone with celiac disease, the good news is that a healthy gut will usually remove all the symptoms that plague you.

IT'S A FACT

According to the National Institute of Health, 5–10 percent of the US population suffers from at least one of the eighty autoimmune diseases currently known.[86]

Probiotics and the Healthy Gut Zone diet (as described in chapter 11) will play a vital part in your gut's restoration. If you have celiac disease, the same gut-friendly diet will be of great value going forward, but be sure and strictly avoid all gluten. Refer to appendix C in the back of the book for foods that contain gluten.

GUT DISEASE 6: ULCERATIVE COLITIS

Another common disease of the gut is ulcerative colitis. Now, there are two sicknesses with the same name that may generate some confusion: colitis and ulcerative colitis. We need to define them before we move on:

- *colitis:* inflammation of the colon (large intestine)
- *ulcerative colitis:* an autoimmune disease that causes chronic inflammation of the colon, ulcer-like holes in the gut wall, and bleeding

They share certain similarities and symptoms, but they are not the same thing. To begin with, here are the symptoms of each.

Symptoms of colitis versus ulcerative colitis

Colitis

The symptoms of colitis and the inflammation it brings to the colon resemble many gut-related sicknesses, making it difficult to diagnose accurately. Common colitis symptoms include the following:

- abdominal pain
- bloating
- chills
- cramping
- diarrhea
- fever[87]

Ulcerative colitis

Ulcerative colitis, on the other hand, is a little easier to diagnose. The symptoms can vary, as the severity also varies per person, and they appear gradually, not suddenly, over time. The usual symptoms are these:

- abdominal pain and cramping
- diarrhea, often with blood or pus
- failure to grow (in children)
- fatigue
- fever
- inability to defecate despite urgency
- rectal bleeding—passing small amounts of blood with stool
- rectal pain
- urgency to defecate
- weight loss[88]

Causes of colitis versus ulcerative colitis

These are severe symptoms. What are the causes?

Colitis

There are many possible causes of colitis, including these:

- allergic reactions
- autoimmune
- exposure to radiation or chemicals
- food poisoning
- infections (bacterial, parasitic)
- inflammatory bowel disease (Crohn's disease, ulcerative colitis)
- ischemic colitis
- lack of blood flow to the intestines
- microscopic colitis[89]

Ulcerative colitis

According to Mayo Clinic, "the exact cause of ulcerative colitis remains unknown." Stress and diet were thought to be the causes, but now these are seen as aggravators instead. Other possibilities scientists are exploring include that it is an immune system malfunction or that it is hereditary (in the genes). But "most people with ulcerative colitis don't have this family history."[90]

Ulcerative colitis is an autoimmune disease and an inflammatory bowel disease (IBD), as is Crohn's disease (gut disease 7). In the US, approximately 7 to 10 out of 100,000 individuals have Crohn's disease, and 80 to 120 out of 100,000 have ulcerative colitis. IBS, on the other hand, affects 15,000 individuals out of every 100,000.[91]

While both Crohn's disease and ulcerative colitis are relatively uncommon, people with these diseases are usually miserable. I have found that they need options and hope because what they hear from most doctors is very discouraging.

IT'S A FACT

IBS (irritable bowel syndrome) is not IBD (inflammatory bowel disease). IBD is a full-blown autoimmune disease.[92]

I've been treating patients with colitis and both IBD diseases (Crohn's and ulcerative colitis) for over thirty years, and I've seen many get healed by first fixing the gut. From my experience, one of the biggest causes of colitis and IBD (both ulcerative colitis and Crohn's disease) is the overuse of antibiotics.

As discussed in greater detail earlier (in chapter 4), antibiotics and medications kill off so many good bacteria that the gut is knocked out of balance. The bad bacteria, which unfortunately are hardier than the good bacteria, overpopulate and travel elsewhere in the GI tract.

Things always take a turn for the worse when bad bacteria are in control. It opens the door, with a leaky gut, for so much inflammation and countless autoimmune diseases. Thankfully, there are answers and ways to turn the tide and beat these inflammatory bowel diseases.

Looking for help

Typically, someone with ulcerative colitis (or Crohn's) is told, "Sorry, but there is no cure." That is genuinely discouraging news! But unless people are willing to do what it takes to get their gut healthy again, I would have to agree with that prognosis.

What are the options? After being diagnosed, patients are usually directed to try to manage the symptoms, dealing with flare-ups and periods of remission.[93] That means trying to control the inflammation, trying to suppress the immune response, taking antibiotics, getting enough liquids to combat diarrhea, and avoiding certain foods.

Biologic therapies are medications that suppress the immune system, reduce inflammation, and can induce remissions and response rates that other medicines cannot achieve in treating inflammatory bowel diseases.[94] The biologic drugs used for IBD include Humira, Remicade, and others that target the tumor necrosis factor alpha (TNF-alpha), which fuels inflammation.[95] This is the usual approach of putting a patch on the problem rather than fixing the core issue, which is the gut.

IT'S A FACT

Ulcerative colitis and Crohn's disease are mostly found in developed countries.[96]

With colitis, living with inflammation in the gut is a nuisance, but for those with ulcerative colitis, they are on the clock. Time is ticking down. If they don't find real answers, they could be looking at a long list of more severe, life-threatening complications, including these:

- blood clots
- colon cancer
- excessive diarrhea causing dehydration
- high blood pressure
- liver damage
- osteoporosis
- skin, eye, and joint inflammation[97]

Some people with ulcerative colitis even reach a point where they need surgery to remove the entire colon. Though this is called a "cure" for ulcerative colitis, the colon is so vital to the body's overall health that its removal is only a last-resort option.[98]

I would never recommend this surgery. Losing your colon would have countless negative ramifications on your gut, metabolism, brain, immune system, and so much more. Thankfully, this is rarely necessary. When you heal the gut, the need for this surgery disappears!

Alternatives/options/choices

With colitis and ulcerative colitis, as with all gut-related sicknesses and disease, I strongly encourage people to get a second opinion from a physician who practices functional medicine.

IT'S A FACT

I prescribe antibiotics for life-threatening diseases. But there is almost always another option along the way. Penicillin, for example, does not have as negative an impact as broad-spectrum antibiotics do. Many antibiotics are prescribed for viral sicknesses and therefore don't have any effect.

No offense, but I have found from decades of experience that most primary care doctors are not thinking about the gut or any of the gut-related diseases. They just don't think that way. They are thinking about a prescription to help with your symptoms and about seeing the next patient in line.

But a healthy gut will usually remove the very symptoms that took you to see the doctor in the first place!

Also, here is a very sobering statistic. Did you know that the fourth leading cause of death in the United States is a severe reaction to the very medications that doctors give their patients?[99]

With colitis and ulcerative colitis, the secret is to restore the gut first. The Healthy Gut Zone diet in chapter 11 outlines the exact steps to restoring your gut. It is an excellent start for colitis and ulcerative colitis. Also, avoid the seven causes of a leaky gut and avoid the ten common enemies of the gut, which were covered in chapters 4 and 6.

A diet high in vegetables, low in carbs and sugar, and high in probiotics has proven extremely helpful for people who have colitis or ulcerative colitis.[100] Because ulcerative colitis is specific to the colon, probiotic enemas can also be especially effective and may be part of the treatment plan. The gut is leaking, and all steps to heal the gut will usually have a positive impact on all gut-related symptoms. Please refer to appendix D for powerful probiotics that can be combined and taken orally or as a probiotic enema.

Despite how annoying colitis is or how threatening ulcerative colitis may be, there are real answers that you can live with. You do not have to be content with patching symptoms. You can heal your gut and live again!

GUT DISEASE 7: CROHN'S DISEASE

Another less common gut issue is Crohn's disease, which is an autoimmune disease that causes inflammation of the entire digestive tract, pain, fatigue, diarrhea, malnutrition, and weight loss. It is an inflammatory bowel disease (IBD), like ulcerative colitis, but can cause damage to any part of the GI tract. While ulcerative colitis is only in the colon, Crohn's can affect the small and large intestines, especially the small intestine and first part of the colon. Oddly enough, severe Crohn's also can affect the skin, joints, eyes, and liver.[101] Researchers estimate that in the US, more than three million people suffer from IBD, which includes Crohn's disease and ulcerative colitis.[102]

IT'S A FACT

People who have Crohn's disease are more sensitive to lectins. Afterall, lectins damage the gut wall.[103]

Symptoms of Crohn's disease

The symptoms of Crohn's disease range from mild to severe, depending on the person and where the disease strikes in the GI tract. As with ulcerative colitis, Crohn's usually develops gradually, though it can come on suddenly. Here are the most common symptoms of Crohn's disease:

- abdominal pain
- blood in your stool
- cramping
- delayed growth or sexual development in children
- diarrhea
- fatigue
- fever
- inflammation of skin, eyes, and joints
- inflammation of the liver or bile ducts
- mouth sores
- pain or drainage near or around the anus due to inflammation from a tunnel into the skin (fistula)
- reduced appetite
- weight loss[104]

And just like ulcerative colitis, if the symptoms persist for a long time, harmful complications are sure to follow. Complications specific to Crohn's disease include these:

- anal fissure (small tear) that may get infected
- anemia (low iron or low B_{12})

- fistulas (ulcers extending through the gut wall, creating a connection between different body parts)
- malnutrition from failure to absorb nutrients
- open sores (ulcers), anywhere from the mouth to anus
- thickening/narrowing of the gut wall, potentially causing blockage[105]

Causes of Crohn's disease

As terribly painful and life-threatening as some of the complications are, what is discouraging is hearing what experts in the medical community say about the cause of Crohn's disease. After all, if you know the cause, you can more easily get to the root of the issue and fix it.

Here are what several foundations, experts, and health communities have to say about the causes of Crohn's:

- "Unfortunately, the causes of Crohn's disease are not yet well understood."[106]
- "The exact cause of Crohn's disease remains unknown."[107]
- "Crohn's disease is an idiopathic condition, which means that scientists aren't yet sure exactly what causes the disease."[108]

Most medical doctors will say the same thing. And because they don't know what causes it, their recommendations for treatments are guesses as well. What are you to do? Again, get a second opinion from a functional medicine physician.

IT'S A FACT

Crohn's disease in teens increased 300 percent in ten years, with junk food and overuse of antibiotics fueling the spike.[109]

Crohn's disease is sometimes caused by a type of bacteria called *Mycobacterium avium subspecies paratuberculosis* (MAP). MAP is widespread in cattle, and as a result, it is found in cheese, milk, and other dairy products. Typically, patients with Crohn's need a culture of fecal tissue to test for MAP.[110]

As with other gut-related diseases, though, I've found one of the biggest causes of Crohn's disease to be the overuse of antibiotics and prescribed medications. Antibiotics and medications (as mentioned in chapter 4) destroy so much of the good bacteria that the bad bacteria take over. Leaky gut naturally follows, as does inflammation and sickness.

For many, the autoimmune disease their bodies will have to address is Crohn's disease. Surgery may be required for Crohn's, but it will not cure the disease because Crohn's is found in so many parts of the GI tract. It is usually almost impossible to cut it out.

There are always answers to beat an autoimmune disease. From symptoms to causes to complications, when the gut is healthy again, everything usually changes for the better.

Alternatives/options/choices

With Crohn's disease, the best remedy is always to work to restore the gut. The Healthy Gut Zone diet in chapter 11 outlines the exact steps to restoring your gut. Also avoid the seven causes of a leaky gut and the ten common enemies of the gut, which were discussed in chapters 4 and 6. This is what I suggest to those who have been diagnosed with Crohn's or have Crohn's symptoms.

IT'S A FACT

People with Crohn's disease and ulcerative colitis need regular colonoscopies.[111]

I usually take patients with Crohn's disease off all dairy and recommend a lot of probiotics and sometimes probiotic enemas. They should strongly consider a fecal transplant as well. See appendix D for probiotics.

Dr. Thomas Borody, an Australian gastroenterologist famous for developing the triple antibiotic therapy for treating *H. pylori* infections, treats many Crohn's and ulcerative colitis patients with fecal transplants from healthy donors.[112] These transplants radically and effectively recolonize the gut with good bacteria.

A few years back, I had a patient with Crohn's disease who traveled on her own to Australia for a fecal transplant. (The FDA in the US allows fecal transplants only for people who suffer from *C. difficile*, a life-threatening and often fatal infection.) When she came back into my offices for a checkup, I could tell something was different. She looked so much healthier. And her Crohn's disease? It was completely gone!

If you would like more information on fecal transplants, please contact my office through the information provided at the end of this book. For most of my patients, however, following the Healthy Gut Zone diet is sufficient to restore their guts, eventually improve and eliminate the symptoms of virtually every autoimmune disease associated with the gut, and put them on the track to health again. And that includes Crohn's disease.

GUT DISEASE 8: BRAIN-RELATED DISEASES

The gut connects to everything. Is it then a stretch of the imagination to think that anxiety, depression, ADHD, and autism can also be linked to the gut? Or that neurodegenerative disorders like Alzheimer's, dementia, and Parkinson's are linked to the gut? Or that obesity is linked to the gut? Or that countless autoimmune diseases are linked to the gut?

IT'S A FACT

About 95 percent of your body's serotonin (good mood chemical) comes from your gut![113]

Believe it or not, all these ailments and diseases are connected to the gut. When you get the gut healthy again, all of this—from the symptoms to the actual diseases—will usually improve and sometimes fade away.

Everything is linked to the health of your gut. Naturally, the physical distance from the gut to the head makes it a bit more difficult to believe there is a strong connection between the GI tract and the brain, but they are more linked than most people realize. The connection is direct—through the vagus nerve.

Cranial nerve X or the vagus nerve runs from the brain stem to the colon. The vagus nerve communicates between your brain and your gut, maintains your heart rate, controls your digestion, regulates various muscles, helps to control your immune system, affects hormones, and much more.[114]

So as you can imagine, in the same way that a leaky gut and bacteria imbalance can hurt your overall health, so it is with your brain. Your gut health has a direct effect on your vagus nerve because it is right there, running from your enteric (intestinal) nervous system to your central nervous system. Of course, nobody would knowingly let anything mess with his or her brain. Yet people do it all the time when they allow their guts to become unhealthy, imbalanced, and leaky.

Let's take a look at several brain-related conditions and how the good and bad bacteria in your gut affect them.

1. Anxiety and depression

Researchers estimate that about forty million adults in the US suffer from anxiety and that women are more than twice as likely than men to experience an anxiety disorder.[115] That is a lot of people battling fear, apprehension, and exaggerated worry! As for depression, about 7 percent (seventeen million) of adults in the US suffer from it per year. Expectedly, "nearly 50 percent of all people diagnosed with depression are also diagnosed with an anxiety disorder."[116]

IT'S A FACT

The foods you eat may treat depression better than antidepressants because the gut is called the "second brain." Treat it well, and it will treat you well.

The gut impacts anxiety and depression. And in reverse, anxiety and depression impact the gut. Consider serotonin, the well-known "good mood" chemical that your body makes. Did you know that approximately 95 percent of the serotonin in your body is made in the gut? And do you know what specifically makes the serotonin? It is the bacteria in your gut.[117]

This is why eating fermented foods and taking probiotics help to reduce anxiety. They boost the good gut bacteria, which in turn make the serotonin and do other tasks for your good gut health. And the more serotonin your body produces, usually the less anxious or depressed you are.

Since the gut makes about 95 percent of the serotonin you enjoy, it's easy to see the connection. Happy gut, better mood! That is a great slogan, and it is 100 percent accurate.

Serotonin is not the only chemical produced when your gut is healthy. Countless others help your body heal, stay healthy, and fight off invaders.

Antidepressants may help with depression, but they do not improve overall brain function, vitality, or enthusiasm. Probiotics improve your body's microbiome, and that has a more significant positive effect.[118]

Remember (from chapter 6) the endotoxin LPS (lipopolysaccharides) that passes between the cells of a damaged gut wall and directly into your bloodstream, causing inflammation all the way to your brain? That inflammation can lead to a long list of sickness, ailments, and autoimmune diseases.

It turns out that depression and inflammation are directly linked and in a very bad way! People with major depression usually have higher LPS levels, which leads to increased gut permeability, chances for becoming obese, and risk of autoimmune diseases and neurodegenerative disorders such as dementia, Alzheimer's, and more.[119]

Probiotics are terrific natural antidepressants.[120]

If you battle anxiety or depression, work on your gut as well. In my opinion, a suggested treatment plan for reducing anxiety and relieving depression should include probiotics. Two documented beneficial probiotics are lactobacilli and bifidobacteria. Probiotics are helpful because they do all of these:

- act like antidepressants[121]
- boost your good gut bacteria[122]
- heal your gut[123]
- help to produce gamma-aminobutyric acid (GABA), which plays a role in emotional balance[124]
- increase serotonin[125]

- lower cytokines[126]
- lower stress[127]
- reduce depression[128]
- turn down (and may turn off) inflammation[129]

In addition to helping with anxiety and depression, probiotics can also improve psychiatric disorder–related behaviors, including autism spectrum disorder, obsessive-compulsive disorder, and memory abilities, including spatial and nonspatial memory.[130]

Combining the Healthy Gut Zone diet in chapter 11 with probiotics is ideal for combatting anxiety and depression.

2. Attention deficit hyperactivity disorder (ADHD)

According to the CDC, the number of children with ADHD jumped by 2–4 percent from 1997 to 2017.[131] As of 2016, around 10 percent of all US children ages four to seventeen had been diagnosed with ADHD, and boys were more than twice as likely to be diagnosed with ADHD as girls. Almost two-thirds of the children are medicated, including children as young as two years of age![132] The usual medication is an amphetamine, which may increase the damage to the gut.

IT'S A FACT

Babies born by C-section are 17 percent more likely to develop ADHD and 33 percent more likely to be diagnosed with autism.[133]

Why the steady increase in ADHD among children? Everything we have talked about in this book—the seven causes of a leaky gut, C-section births and lack of breastfeeding, the typical high-sugar, high-carb diet, and the nine other enemies of the gut—plays a part. It all comes down to the gut.

Carefully consider the words of Dr. Perlmutter: "ADHD is simply a manifestation of inflammation gone awry due to triggers like gluten and the downstream effects of a sick microbiome."[134]

The connection from the gut to the brain is established, and age is no boundary. The fact that young children can have brain-related issues because of a gut out of order is a scary thought—not only for them but also for us!

Two very beneficial probiotics (lactobacilli and bifidobacteria) produce necessary chemicals that help the body, including GABA.[135] It is this GABA that helps us keep our emotions balanced. And children with ADHD? Their brains have very little GABA![136]

GABA production needs zinc and vitamin B_6 from the foods we eat (or should be eating). But even if we are eating enough of the right foods or taking supplements with zinc or B_6 (which few are), the gut usually cannot adequately absorb vitamins from food if the gut is impaired.

Thankfully, in regard to ADHD, probiotics are particularly effective in boosting GABA levels.[137] Couple that with a healthy diet, rather than medications, and the body will steadily improve.

I recommend that children with ADHD get off gluten, excessive sugars, and artificial food coloring or dyes right away. That alone will often reduce inflammation and its adverse effects on the body and brain considerably. The Healthy Gut Zone diet in chapter 11 is a natural next step to treat ADHD.

3. Autism spectrum disorder

Autism spectrum disorder (ASD) includes other conditions that used to be diagnosed separately, such as autistic disorder, pervasive developmental disorder not otherwise specified (PDD-NOS), and Asperger's syndrome.[138] All of these are considered ASD now.

Research shows that one in fifty-four children in the US have ASD. From 2000 to 2016, in just sixteen years, the rate of children diagnosed with ASD almost tripled![139]

IT'S A FACT

"More than 3.5 million Americans live with an autism spectrum disorder,"[140] and this number keeps growing. It affects boys about four times more than girls.[141]

Interestingly, the most common GI tract complaints from those with autism are constipation, diarrhea, and heartburn.[142] I used to wonder why gut issues would be prevalent with a more mental issue such as ASD, but it makes complete sense when you look at things from the perspective that the gut is central to the problem. For decades, doctors have been studying the connection between ASD and the gut. They have found that as many as 70 percent of those with ASD also have gut issues.[143]

Many factors may cause ASD. It is not just a single thing. A leaky gut, unhealthy diet, and antibiotics will certainly play a part, but so will all the components connected to a leaky gut and the microbiome.[144]

Healing the gut is a big part of the equation because of its direct link to the brain. Dr. Raphael Kellman boldly states, "We can actually change the conversations that produce brain dysfunction, and we can change them at their source."[145] The "source" is the gut.

IT'S A FACT

As with depression, LPS levels are usually high with those who have severe autism,[146] and that means massive inflammation in the entire body, including the brain.

Again, probiotics are a great help. They may help reduce autistic behavior. I have even seen some pretty incredible results with a family who chose fecal transplants for their son. Within a month, the gut bacteria changed from being imbalanced to the bad to being imbalanced to the good, and the autistic behavior problems were dramatically reduced. It was incredible.

ASD affects how the brain processes information, and that is readily apparent in times of social interaction. When the gut is healthy, the neurotransmitters are more likely to be balanced, which gives the body far more control than is typical. The difference is usually astounding.

Now, these treatments can help, but I do not say that they are cures. Why not? Because everyone with autism has different symptoms, different severity levels, and different levels of gut health.

With that said, autism patients have a good chance of seeing improvement, regardless of their situation, age, or condition, when they work to restore their gut health. It is that effective because everything connects to the gut.

4. Alzheimer's, dementia, and Parkinson's

The three most common brain-related diseases are Alzheimer's (the most common type of dementia), dementia (Lewy body dementia [LBD], frontotemporal dementia [FTD], vascular dementia, etc.), and Parkinson's disease. Alzheimer's disease and other forms of dementia are fatal, often through an agonizingly slow, expensive, and increasingly debilitating process. Although Parkinson's itself isn't fatal, its complications can be.[147] All have stages that are measured as mild, moderate, or severe. If you or anyone you know has one of these diseases, the best hope for treatment is to address it early, especially if it is in the "pre" stages.

IT'S A FACT

Usually, a leaky gut eventually leads to a leaky brain. Never forget that.

- Alzheimer's usually affects people over age sixty-five, and about 10 percent of the US older population has Alzheimer's. Of these, nearly two-thirds are women.[148]

- Dementia affects a larger number of people, but 60–80 percent of those who have dementia suffer from Alzheimer's disease.[149]

- Parkinson's is the second most common neurodegenerative disorder after Alzheimer's, with about sixty thousand new diagnoses each year in the US.[150]

And they are all connected to the gut? Absolutely! Often, inflammation and a leaky gut eventually lead to a leaky brain. And anything that causes or perpetuates inflammation, such as the foods we eat, can eventually lead to a leaky brain. The natural blood/brain barrier keeps toxins out of the brain, but that barrier is not as impenetrable as we once believed. Small molecules *can* and *do* leak through![151]

Recent studies are finding that the bacteria in your gut can make the blood/brain barrier more permeable (leaky) to microbes.[152] It's not the good bacteria doing this! It's the gram-negative bacteria and the LPS that protect these bacteria from digestion that cause a significant inflammatory response and therefore a leaky gut and a leaky brain.[153] We now know that Alzheimer's patients have three times as much LPS in their plasma as healthy people.[154]

A diet of saturated fats, such as butter, cheese, cream, coconut oil, and fatty meats, increases the body's absorption of LPS.[155] All this information shouts out just how important the bacteria balance in the gut is and why we need to lower our saturated fat intake.

Also vitally important in the fight against Alzheimer's, dementia, and Parkinson's is the need for stopping inflammation and restoring a leaky gut. Those are two immediate and vital steps that must be taken. Go to the source and drastically change your diet. Usually, by so doing, you decrease the inflammation in the brain, which minimizes further damage.

The Healthy Gut Zone diet in chapter 11 will become your friend. In addition to knowing what foods to avoid, it will be helpful to know which foods are beneficial. Polyphenols found in cocoa, coffee, and curcumin are specifically beneficial for protecting the brain.

Another element that must be controlled (and the Healthy Gut Zone diet does this) is blood sugar levels. Consuming excessive sugar feeds brain-related diseases. The gut is not only at the center of elevated blood sugar levels, but it is also at the center of brain disease.[156]

Elevated blood sugar levels from eating a lot of carbohydrates, sugars, or starches trigger glycation. (Glycation is the binding of sugars to proteins and causes damage to many tissues and organs.) This, in turn, can damage nerves, the brain, eyes, blood vessels, kidneys, and skin. Glycation will actually accelerate your aging process![157]

But that is not all. The brain can itself become glycated, with brain cells that become glycated or cross-linked (sugars irregularly bonding to proteins) because of the excessive sugars. Glycated tissues and organs are damaged and undergo accelerated aging, and memory usually worsens.

That is why people with type 2 diabetes are so much more likely to get Alzheimer's or dementia. Their imbalanced sugar levels and insulin resistance lead right into the inflammation that feeds these brain-related diseases.[158]

It now makes complete sense why sugar levels, right up there with inflammation and leaky gut, play such a significant role in your body's health from head to toe. In my opinion, the absolute best defense against Alzheimer's, dementia, and Parkinson's is to have a healthy gut, plain and simple. The Healthy Gut Zone diet will do just that.

5. Obesity

According to the CDC, obesity rates keep climbing, despite all the new diets, health scares, and knowledge that we throw at it. Year after year, it gets only worse. Currently, about 42 percent of the US population is obese.[159] The World Health Organization classifies obesity as one of the top five most significant health risks in modern societies.[160]

IT'S A FACT

"Being overweight or obese significantly increases the chances of cognitive decline, loss of brain tissue, and...various brain diseases, from depression to dementia." It also increases your risk of diabetes, heart disease, inflammation, and much more.[161]

Sadly, obesity (that is, a body mass index of 30 or higher for an adult) leads directly to at least twenty-five other health conditions, including thirteen different cancers![162] And believe it or not, one study estimated the health-care cost to handle these numbers of obese people at about $190 billion per year![163] Being obese is an incredibly dangerous and frightfully expensive position to be in, and yet it is an entirely preventable epidemic.

Wait! Don't our genes determine obesity? Not entirely. It may have much less to do with our genes and much more to do with our guts!

What role does the gut play with obesity? First of all, the Healthy Gut Zone diet will usually stop obesity dead in its tracks. By staying in the Healthy Gut Zone, most people lose weight, and many may overcome obesity. There are countless diets and exercise regimens to choose from, but if you are looking to lose weight and get your gut healthy again, I suggest the Healthy Gut Zone diet.

Second of all, the gut plays an increasingly important role in our metabolism. Consider the ongoing battle of dominance between the good and bad bacteria in your gut. Did you know that the food cravings we blame on a lack of willpower might be the result of bad bacteria in the gut? Consider this statement by Dr. Robynne Chutkan:

> Gut bacteria are able to influence our food choices by releasing molecules that affect our brain, including hormones like serotonin

that affect mood and make us feel good after eating certain foods. They can even change the properties of taste receptors so that particular flavors are more or less satisfying to our palate.[164]

In other words, the bad bacteria in your gut could very well be making you want to eat the foods you should not be eating! True, we are all responsible for our actions, but when the body and brain gang up on us and tell us what to eat, it is admittedly very hard to resist.

Why does the gut have such control? The answer once again is in the balance of bacteria. Have you ever gone without sugar or carbs for a period of time, usually a week or two, and then noticed that your desire for those foods was significantly reduced? That is what I am talking about. When good bacteria gain control in the gut, you naturally want healthier foods. And if the bad bacteria are in control, they want the foods that feed them, which is precisely the high-sugar, high-carb diet.

IT'S A FACT

The higher the number of Firmicutes in your gut, the higher your risk for sickness, disease, inflammation, and weight gain.[165]

As you know, what you eat determines what bacteria grow in your gut. Now we know that those same bacteria, good or bad, can talk back to you, pressuring you to eat the foods that will provide more growth for them.

Ask yourself this simple question: What foods am I craving?

What came to mind? Regardless of the time of day, cravings are usually a clear sign of the bacteria in your gut talking to you. What are they saying?

But it is not all about wanting foods. It is also about what happens to those foods when they get into your GI tract. When someone is obese, he or she has a higher ratio of bad than good bacteria in the gut. One bacteria type, in particular, stands out as perhaps the greatest cause of weight gain of all, and those are Firmicutes.

What do these nasty Firmicutes do that is so bad? Firmicutes cause your body to pull more calories from what you eat, thus making your food more caloric. This directly causes you to gain weight.[166]

Two people can eat the same food and get different results. It doesn't seem fair! A healthy person with a healthy gut, and thus lower Firmicute levels, can eat the same thing that an overweight or obese person with higher Firmicute levels might eat, and the healthy person doesn't gain weight while the obese or overweight person does.

As we noted in chapter 1, Firmicutes and Bacteroidetes—bad and good bacteria, respectively—account for most of the bacteria in your gut. The ratio between the two determines our tendency for

- diseases,
- inflammation,
- metabolism, and
- weight gain.[167]

No exact ratio of Firmicutes to Bacteroidetes fits everyone. But generally, the fewer Firmicutes, the better.

In a 2013 study, researchers transferred fecal matter from sets of human twins, where one twin was obese and the other slender, into lean mice to populate the mice's gut microbiome. The body fat and mass of mice who received bacteria from the obese human twins increased significantly. But mice who received bacteria from the slender human twins and who ate a healthy diet stayed lean. The obese mice had a higher ratio of Firmicutes to Bacteroidetes compared to the leaner mice.[168]

IT'S A FACT

Craving sugary, starchy foods? It could be yeast overgrowth (SIFO).[169]

Now, other factors are involved in weight management, such as caloric intake, exercise routines, muscle mass, metabolic rate, eating and drinking habits, sickness, and others. Still, the point in all this is that the gut needs to be healthy. With a healthy gut, the bacteria are usually in the proper ratio, and that is necessary and beneficial to anyone trying to lose weight.

Your gut bacteria balance is a snapshot of where you are going as well as where you currently are. Scientists are now able to look at the bacteria in your gut and predict your risk of becoming obese with 80–90 percent accuracy.[170]

That is great news! By now, you know that it is possible to change the bacteria ratio in your gut. When you put the good bacteria in charge, everything turns out for the better. It also makes losing weight so much easier!

Over the years, I have witnessed thousands of people defeat obesity, and those who lost the weight and kept it off usually did so by getting their gut healthy again. That is where every weight-loss program needs to begin.

Alternatives/options/choices

With all these brain-related conditions, ailments, and diseases, good gut health is the best answer. It is not only a great defense; it is also an incredible offense. It is the foundation of all good health as well as the wettest blanket on the raging fires of inflammation. It is always the best thing you can do to get your health back.

Some studies show that if you fix a leaky gut, then you could reverse the gut's autoimmune response and roll back the symptoms that cause so much damage.[171] Granted, it's not all about a leaky gut or about inflammation. Still, after you stop a leaky gut and stop inflammation, I would be very interested in what symptoms, ailments, or diseases you will have left. I can't say it enough: the best sign of a healthy body is a healthy gut.

IT'S A FACT

Good gut bacteria help to turn off or decrease inflammation.

GUT DISEASE 9: AUTOIMMUNE DISEASES

As you know, about 70–80 percent of your immune system is in your gut.[172] The immune system holds bacteria in the mucus of the GI tract—a short but safe distance from the gut wall—until it is processed as bad (and killed and swept out) or good (and allowed to stay).[173] But if the gut wall is leaky, permeable, or weakened for one of many reasons, then anything that gets through the gut wall without official immune system approval will be seen as an enemy that must be destroyed.

This overactive immune system is most often the cause of massive inflammation, but it can eventually cause an autoimmune attack. Your body is unknowingly attacking itself, all because things are getting through the gut wall!

The many autoimmune diseases are based on the commonality of the body fighting against itself. But that is not the only common trait about autoimmune diseases. Did you also know this?

- All autoimmune diseases involve inflammation.
- Autoimmune diseases usually have the same root cause: a leaky gut.
- A healthy gut typically helps improve all diseases.

There are more than eighty different autoimmune diseases.[174] Here is a sampling:

- Addison's disease
- alopecia areata
- ankylosing spondylitis
- celiac disease
- Crohn's disease
- dermatomyositis
- diabetes (type 1)
- eczema
- eosinophilic esophagitis
- Graves' disease
- Hashimoto's thyroiditis
- immune thrombocytopenic purpura (ITP)
- interstitial cystitis
- juvenile arthritis
- lupus
- multiple sclerosis (MS)
- myasthenia gravis
- polymyositis

- primary biliary cirrhosis
- primary sclerosing cholangitis
- psoriasis
- psoriatic arthritis
- Raynaud's phenomenon
- rheumatoid arthritis
- sarcoidosis
- scleroderma
- Sjögren's syndrome
- ulcerative colitis
- urticaria
- vasculitis
- vitiligo

An estimated 23.5 million Americans suffer from at least one autoimmune disease.[175]

Alternatives/options/choices

The best treatment will be the same for any autoimmune disease: get your gut healthy again. Boost the good bacteria in your GI tract, as that alone may turn off the autoimmune system response. Probiotics will usually help.

IT'S A FACT

Avoiding lectins has been found to cure autoimmune diseases.[176]

If you have an autoimmune disease, get on the Healthy Gut Zone diet as quickly as you can. The relief you find on this diet may be so significant that you will want to stay there indefinitely. And if it makes life better, it's an excellent place to be.

PART III
GUT ANSWERS

PART 3 IS full of answers. It provides you with the Healthy Gut Zone diet outline and the practical steps you can take to get your gut back to a healthy state. This is where your gut wants to go, and now you have the tools to get you there.

CHAPTER NINE

PREPARING FOR YOUR JOURNEY

WHY ARE YOU looking for answers? Are you facing health challenges? Would your body significantly improve if your gut was healthy again?

Suffering from any ailment, sickness, or disease is the worst. When I had psoriasis, it almost drove me crazy! I fought it daily for years. On top of that, it was embarrassing. My patients wondered how I could help them since I could not seem to help myself! The answer for my psoriasis was far less complicated, far less expensive, and far less intrusive than I ever imagined. And once my gut and I quit fighting each other, my psoriasis cleared up!

Perhaps you are here because you or someone you love is battling one of the not-so-friendly sicknesses or diseases we've been discussing in this book. I have seen so many lives radically changed for the better as a result of people applying the principles of the Healthy Gut Zone diet. It is impossible, of course, to guarantee anything in the medical profession. Still, I will say that I am no longer surprised when people tell me their "irreversible" disease, diagnosis, or situation is much improved or completely eradicated after they got their gut healthy again.

Fantastic health benefits are realized when the gut heals itself. As the foundation to so much, whether good or bad, the gut plays a surprisingly pivotal role in basically every disease known to man. In short, a healthy gut can usher in health and healing, literally from head to toe.

So, regardless of why you are here, let's get your gut healthy again. Then you can see what happens after that!

GET READY TO START BY STOPPING

One of the most important steps on your journey to gut health is to immediately stop eating, drinking, or doing whatever it is that harms your GI tract. Only by removing the things that cause the inflammation and leaky gut are you able to break your body free from the cycle it is in. Remember, the body usually craves the very foods that invite inflammation and disease into the body.

IT'S A FACT

You don't need to be pregnant for alcohol to be bad for you because alcohol is not gut friendly.

> *» Alcohol can increase inflammation in the gut.*
> *» Alcohol lowers your immunity levels.*
> *» Alcohol can cause bowel irritation.*
> *» Alcohol can increase the craving for more.*
> *» Alcohol can feed bad bacteria.[1]*

Here is my list of things you should try to avoid:

- alcohol (best to remove entirely)
- antibiotics
- anti-inflammatory medications (such as aspirin, Advil, Motrin, Aleve, etc.)
- artificial sweeteners
- chlorinated water
- dairy (cheese, milk, cream, butter, yogurt, etc.)
- excessive meats, especially processed meats and fatty meats
- gluten
- GMO foods

- high-lectin foods (usually can add some back in two to three months—more on this later)*
- medications for GERD and acid-blocking meds
- processed foods (most foods in a box) and excessive starches and carbs (potatoes, rice, corn). Limit starches to the size of a tennis ball and only one per meal (if over eighteen).
- saturated fats (reduce or eliminate), especially butter, cheese, cream, and coconut oil
- sugar
- Some may need to switch from fluoride toothpaste to a natural toothpaste since fluoride kills good bacteria if swallowed, or rinse their mouths out well after using a fluoride toothpaste.

Technically, everything on this list pretty much damages the gut, contributes to inflammation in the gut, or gives the bad bacteria in your gut a boost. You don't want that.

IT'S A FACT

Fiber, probiotics, prebiotics, and polyphenols are four of your gut's best friends.

This list will probably not cure anything, but it usually does have an immediate or almost-immediate effect on the symptoms that patients have. You want to feed only the good bacteria because those are working on your side to make your body healthy. Stopping what feeds the bad bacteria is a perfect first step.

ADD THE RIGHT NUTRIENTS TO YOUR GUT

Restoring your gut is not a supplement-heavy endeavor because removing the meds and gut-damaging foods is the key to healing your gut. You are

---

* However, children and teens (those less than eighteen years of age) should consume adequate healthy starches and carbohydrates. We will discuss this more later.

not going to be buying bottles and bottles of expensive exotic herbs or supplements. It's not necessary.

Your gut needs the right nutrients so that it can heal. Some of this will come from a few supplements, but most will be the result of eating foods that have what your gut needs.

IT'S A FACT

Polyphenols are phytonutrients in certain plants that boost your immune system, strengthen your entire GI tract, and help your brain function properly. Foods and beverages rich in polyphenols include certain olive oils, cocoa powder, dark chocolate, berries, chestnuts, cloves, and coffee.

The overall goal is for your gut to regain the proper balance of good bacteria, stamp out the bad microbes, heal the holes in the gut wall, and quench inflammation in the gut. To achieve this, you will usually need to include these things in your diet:

- fiber
- polyphenols
- prebiotics
- probiotics

Depending on your symptoms, ailments, or disease, supplements such as the following will be of additional and specific value:

- BPC 157 peptide (a peptide to help restore a leaky gut)
- colostrum (to repair leaky gut) if not sensitive to dairy
- deglycyrrhizinated licorice (DGL; to repair leaky gut)
- herbs (slippery elm, marshmallow root, and aloe vera to soothe and protect the gut and boost mucus production)
- hydrolyzed collagen (to help repair leaky gut)
- L-glutamine (to help repair leaky gut)

- magnesium (to improve bowel motility)
- omega-3 (to help quench inflammation and repair the gut)
- vitamin D$_3$ (to help regulate gut bacteria)
- zinc (to improve the barrier function of the gut)

You will even need to start (if you don't already) eating some foods that are incredibly beneficial to the good bacteria in your gut, such as these:

- fermented foods
- resistant starches

Thankfully, your gut will usually heal itself when you feed it the right foods and remove whatever has been causing problems. The process is amazingly simple.

You may not be able to eat or drink some of the foods and beverages you want, or you may have to reduce them significantly, but your gut health and your overall body's health depend on getting your gut strong again. It is certainly worth it!

UNDERSTAND THE SIGNS

There are some things in life that you probably don't want to learn about but that can be helpful to know. Poop is one of those things.

IT'S A FACT

Heal the lining of the gut and food sensitivities usually go away.

It seemed strange at first, but I quickly learned that most of my patients in their seventies and eighties are always talking about their bowel movements. Now, as you know, constipation is a common problem and the cause of many doctor visits. When you fix their constipation, they are always delighted! They also feel great, and that only fuels more conversations about poop.

Constipation usually worsens with age. The mixture of inadequate water intake, aging muscles, medications (especially antacids), and a low-fiber diet impact millions of people every year in the US.

How you sit on the toilet also plays a part. Did you know that "hemorrhoids, digestive diseases like diverticulitis, and even constipation are common only in countries where people generally sit on some kind of chair [or toilet] to pass their stool"?[2]

When pooping, you have two sphincter muscles (and two nervous systems) that work together, one at the end (the anus) and another just inside the first. You can control the outer muscle, but the inner one is automatic. The inner sphincter muscle opens first, then the outer (anus) sphincter when stools are passed.[3]

The fastest position for pooping is squatting. It is easier on your GI tract and your colon in particular, and that causes you less strain. The typical sitting position on a toilet causes a slight kink in the colon, and that slows down the process. It also makes for more straining and pushing.

Your colon is one continuous intestine made up of three distinct parts:

- ascending colon
- transverse colon
- descending colon (including the sigmoid colon and rectum)

Think of each part holding your food for one day, which makes the full cycle a three-day routine. Typically, what you ate for breakfast on Monday is in your ascending colon throughout the day, your transverse colon on Tuesday, and then your descending colon on Wednesday. When you do go to the bathroom, you empty only the descending colon or last third of your colon.[4]

More information about poop that you never wanted to know or talk about includes the following:

- Poop composition: Poop is three-fourths water. The last fourth is made of bacteria, indigestible vegetable fiber, and body waste (medicines, food coloring, cholesterol, etc.).[5]

- Laxatives and enemas: Taking a laxative or using an enema may empty your entire colon. It will usually take you three days to refill again.[6]

- Poop chart: Maybe you have seen the Bristol Stool Chart.[7] It describes the different types of poop:

Type 1

Separate hard lumps, like nuts
(hard to pass)

Type 2

Sausage-shaped but lumpy

Type 3

Like a sausage but with cracks
on its surface

Type 4

Like a sausage or snake,
smooth and soft

Type 5

Soft blobs with clear-cut edges
(passed easily)

Type 6

Fluffy pieces with ragged edges,
a mushy stool

Type 7

Watery, no solid pieces;
entirely liquid

- Best poop type: Maybe you are wondering, based on achieving a healthy gut, which of these seven stool types is the best to have. I recommend stool types 3, 4, and 5. All are easy to pass, and it means you have a good flow (about three days), ample liquids, and sufficient fiber.

- Wiping: It may surprise you (perhaps not), but when the colon is in a good cycle (producing stool types 3, 4, or 5), you will hardly even need to wipe. If a lot of toilet paper is necessary, something is often wrong. Usually, you need more fiber and probiotics, magnesium, or water. Needing to use very little toilet paper is a sign that your poop is good.

- Pooping stool: I recommend a small footstool (such as a Squatty Potty) about six to eight inches tall that you can slide under your feet when you are sitting on the toilet. This position will decrease pressure, maintain the best colon position, and make pooping a whole lot easier on your body.

- Gas: Almost all foods and drinks create gas (nitrogen, oxygen, hydrogen, carbon dioxide, and methane) in your colon as a natural result of the fermenting process. Too much gas is usually the result of eating such things as sugars (including lactose from dairy and fructose from fruits), beans, peas, lentils, broccoli, peanuts, cashews, carbs, cruciferous veggies, and starches. To decrease gas, drink more water, eat/drink less of what causes gas, and take sufficient probiotics. A lot of gas is a sign of excessive fermenting, whether it's what you ate or a symptom of another gut-related ailment such as SIBO or SIFO. Patients with SIBO and SIFO should take caution with fiber. Start low at one-quarter teaspoon a day, and go slow.

What might be messing with your colon and causing constipation? The most common causes I see include these:

- lack of exercise
- lack of fiber
- lack of fluids
- lack of magnesium

- sluggish or low thyroid
- too much stress

Most people fail to drink enough water (at least eight cups per day, although more fluid intake is recommended[8]), yet drinking adequate water is easy enough to do.

IT'S A FACT

How long should it take to poop? "Most professionals recommend spending no more time on the toilet than it takes to pass a stool. Studies have shown the average bowel movement takes 12 seconds."[9]

As for fiber and magnesium, we seldom get enough of these in the foods we eat, which means taking them as supplements is the only other option. Adult Americans eat 15–16 grams of fiber a day on average.[10] The USDA recommends for adults under fifty years of age to consume 25–28 grams a day of fiber for women and 31–34 grams a day for men. If over age fifty, it is 22 grams for women and 28 grams for men.[11]

I have found that most of my patients are deficient in both fiber and magnesium. Odds are, you are low as well. Approximately 50 percent of the US population is deficient in magnesium.[12] You can increase your magnesium intake by eating foods such as spinach, kale, almonds, dark chocolate, and avocados, which are also gut friendly. One ounce of almonds contains 80 milligrams of magnesium. Other magnesium-rich foods that are not gut friendly include whole wheat, black beans, and edamame. The recommended daily allowance (RDA) for magnesium is 310–420 milligrams for adults, depending on age and gender.[13]

IT'S A FACT

Fecal transplants are the transferring of stool from a healthy person to the infected person's colon (the rectum and sigmoid in the descending colon area). Most often this is administered as an enema, but it can also be in a pill form that the person swallows as part of a regimen that lasts for several days. The FDA allows the use of fecal transplants only to treat C. difficile. Still, other countries use fecal transplants to treat other gut-related sicknesses and diseases, including Crohn's disease and ulcerative colitis. Fecal transplants are meant to provide a massive boost to the GI tract's good bacteria.

Add in some probiotics and prebiotics, and you are well on your way to healing your gut.

GET USED TO EATING HEALTHY FOODS

Eating to keep your gut happy and healthy is not as foreign, difficult, or freaky as many might think. Here are some of the natural foods that are great for your diet:

- **Avocado**—This is probably the absolute best fruit/vegetable (a fruit that we use as a veggie) that was ever grown. Most fruits are full of sugar, and sugar feeds the bad bacteria in your gut, but an avocado is almost sugar free. It also has good fats (avocado oil is very good for you) and fiber (most people are low in fiber) and contains magnesium and potassium. Avocados cause some with IBS and SIBO to have more gas, since avocados are a high FODMAP food, so start low and go slow.

- **Oils**—Organic, extra-virgin avocado and olive oils are full of vitamins, minerals, and polyphenols. Your gut needs all of these nutrients all the time. Use both of these oils liberally on your foods at any meal. Olive oil reduces inflammation,[14] and the polyphenols in olive oil help to heal the gut.

- **Greens**—You will be eating a lot of salads, so get a range of greens. Veggies such as romaine lettuce, red and green leaf lettuce, arugula, field greens, kohlrabi, mesclun (baby greens), spinach, endive, butter lettuce, parsley, fennel, and seaweed/sea vegetables are also lectin free,[15] which is ideal for your gut. Apply liberal amounts of avocado or olive oil.

- **Resistant starches**—Instead of the usual white or red potatoes, shift to sweet potatoes, yucca, or taro root, but limit to a
  half cup per serving because they are high in carbs. These are
  full of what your gut wants: not much sugar and lots of fiber,
  vitamins, and minerals.

- **Lean, grass-fed, grass-finished meat and wild low-mercury
  fish**—Meat is an excellent source of protein, but too much of
  it can slow down your digestion process. As you know, your
  gut needs gut-friendly foods, so find meats that are wild (i.e.,
  fish), organic range-fed (i.e., chicken and turkey), and grass-fed
  and grass-finished (i.e., beef), and wild low-mercury fish, such
  as wild Alaskan salmon, tongol tuna, sardines, wild flounder,
  wild tilapia, wild cod, wild herring, and haddock. Think two-
  thirds veggies and one-fourth to one-third meat (two to three
  ounces for women, three to six ounces for men) at meals. Avoid
  processed meats, such as bacon, sausage, pepperoni, salami,
  and others.

- **Starches**—Instead of bread, pasta, corn, and rice, choose
  millet bread or bread made from almond flour, coconut flour,
  or cassava flour, or tortillas from cassava. (See appendix A.)

Your gut wants you to think this way:

- Feed me foods low in sugars and low in carbs that are also
  full of fiber, probiotics, prebiotics, and polyphenols, and I will
  be happy.

- If I am happy, you are healthy.

- And if you are healthy, you are happy.

That is the underlying goal when it comes to choosing foods, eating healthfully, and nourishing your gut. It should not be too complicated or too difficult. If it is, nobody will do it. Thankfully, the gut is pretty easy to please.

IT'S A FACT

Here are the terms to look for when purchasing the gut-friendliest meats:

- » *Chicken: You want* pastured, organic, *or* free-range (not soy or corn fed).
- » *Beef: You want* grass-fed *and* grass-finished.
- » *Fish: You want it* wild *or* wild-caught (not farm-raised).

My book *Dr. Colbert's Keto Zone Diet* is a great place to start. Just decrease or eliminate saturated fats, including butter, cheese, coconut oil and cream, and fatty meats. (MCT oil is a safe and healthy saturated fat and does not raise LPS levels like coconut oil.) Increase your good gut-healing carbs such as sweet potatoes, yams, yucca, taro root, cassava, jicama, and millet bread to about 35–100 grams a day of total carb intake. A small sweet potato has approximately 27 grams of carbs, one slice of millet bread has approximately 21 grams, a half cup taro root has 14 grams of carbs, and one cup of jicama has only 11 grams of carbs. Recipes typically have about 20–25 grams of healthy carbs per meal, which is usually one slice of millet bread or a half cup of most of the carbs mentioned previously. Lime cassava chips are an excellent snack with avocado or guacamole.

CHAPTER TEN

FIVE GUT POWER TOOLS FOR YOUR GUT HEALTH

PATIENTS COME INTO my offices all the time who are suffering from one symptom or another. With fifty patients, we could easily be talking about five hundred different symptoms, and usually, each patient is already taking one or more different prescriptions. That's the norm.

But another norm may be of interest. If all the patients would work to restore their gut health and eat the same gut-friendly foods, including fiber, probiotics, prebiotics, and polyphenols, most likely every single person would see improvement. Most symptoms would likely disappear and any sicknesses and diseases along with them.

That is how powerful the gut is. Once it is restored, it can put the rest of your body back together again! If you are looking to improve your gut health, the following pages outline five powerful tools—*gut power tools*—that are proven to be incredibly good for your gut.

Gut Power Tool 1: Fiber

The first gut power tool is plain old fiber—not beans, wheat bran, or grain-based fibers that are full of lectins but psyllium husk powder. Not very exciting or cool, but it plays an amazingly vital role in restoring your gut health. It is also very inexpensive, which makes it available to everyone.

You might be wondering why fiber is all that special. It is, after all, a natural ingredient in many fruits, legumes, and vegetables. It's all around us, so why is it so valuable?

To begin with, very few people get enough fiber in their diet. Rarely is a single one of my patients getting sufficient fiber. In fact, only 5 percent of Americans have an adequate intake of fiber.[1]

Because most of our society is low in fiber, it is then not surprising at all to see common low-fiber symptoms show up everywhere. Here are five common symptoms most people experience without sufficient fiber intake:

1. constipation, which could lead to hemorrhoids, anal fissures, and diverticulosis and diverticulitis

2. inability to lose weight and easy weight gain

3. low energy (feeling sluggish and lethargic)

4. hungry soon after eating

5. craving between meals[2]

Total surprise, right? I mean, how often do people complain about constipation, fatigue, or the failure to lose weight? All the time! As you very well know, constipation is one of the most common reasons for doctor visits. And fatigue and not being able to lose weight—those apply to almost everyone on the planet!

Of course, you can't blame everything on fiber, for it is just one of the many different pieces of the healthy-gut puzzle. Unfortunately, most of the high-fiber foods that people eat are whole wheat based, and that usually damages the gut.

The many benefits of fiber

At a glance, the many benefits of fiber may be surprising. Did you know that fiber

- helps to control blood sugar levels,
- may lower blood pressure,
- lowers cholesterol,
- makes you feel full longer, causing you to reduce food intake and lose weight,
- usually normalizes bowel movements,
- lowers risk of heart disease,
- minimizes hemorrhoids, and
- may help prevent diverticular disease?[3]

With those lists of benefits, it is understandable if you now no longer want to run low on daily fiber intake! I recommend 30–35 grams of fiber per day, but start low and go slow to avoid bloating and gas.

Getting enough fiber

Technically, fiber comes in two different forms: soluble and insoluble. Your body needs both.

Soluble fiber dissolves in your GI tract, absorbs water, and helps with digestion. As you see below, most of these fibers are typically not gut friendly.

Sources of soluble fiber include these:

- apples (usually not gut friendly)
- barley (usually not gut friendly)
- beans (usually not gut friendly unless pressure-cooked)
- carrots (usually gut friendly)
- citrus fruits (lemons and limes are fine, but others are high in sugar)
- oats (usually not gut friendly)
- peas (usually not gut friendly unless pressure-cooked)
- psyllium (usually gut friendly)[4]

Insoluble fiber does not dissolve in your GI tract. It passes through, helps keep you regular, and pushes food through the GI tract.

Sources of insoluble fiber include the following:

- beans (usually not gut friendly unless pressure-cooked)
- cauliflower (usually gut friendly, but be careful with gas)
- green beans (usually not gut friendly unless pressure-cooked)
- nuts (usually gut friendly, but not peanuts or cashews)
- potatoes (usually not gut friendly)
- wheat bran (not gut friendly)
- whole-wheat flour (not gut friendly)[5]

Based on what we have discussed throughout this book, you may be wondering if the lectins, gluten, starches, or sugars in these soluble and insoluble fiber sources are okay to eat to get sufficient amounts of fiber you need. That is a good question!

IT'S A FACT

The fiber in your food makes you feel more satisfied after you eat it.[6]

My answer is probably what you are already thinking as well:

- Eating fruit to get fiber means eating fruit sugars, and any sugar feeds the bad bacteria in your gut. So for the next few months at least, I would not recommend fiber from fruit, except for berries (one-quarter to one-half cup a day), which are low in sugar and high in polyphenols. Carrots and apples also have sugar, though it is much less than in citrus fruits.

- Eating beans, peas, barley, whole wheat, wheat bran, and potatoes to get fiber means eating lectins, gluten, and starch. That is not good for your gut wall. Pressure-cooking beans and peas properly to remove lectins, after one or two months of avoidance, is a good plan, but I would stay away completely from gluten. So for the next few months, I would get your fiber from other sources, such as veggies, berries, and perhaps psyllium husk powder, if you do not experience gas or bloating.

How then do you get enough fiber? My top recommendation for soluble fiber intake is psyllium husk powder. Psyllium is mainly a soluble fiber with some insoluble fiber from the seed husks of the plant Plantago ovata.

Many laxative or fiber mixes claim to provide your body with the fiber it needs. Though that might be true, it is the other ingredients (especially sugars and artificial sweeteners) that concern me. You can buy the psyllium husk powder by itself, with nothing else added to it. It is inexpensive and available online and in most health-food stores, but do not buy the psyllium husk powder with sugar, NutraSweet, or Splenda. (For those who dislike the taste, we have a great-tasting, healthy fiber listed in appendix D.)

The amount you want to start with on a regular daily basis is one-quarter teaspoon of psyllium husk powder in a four-ounce glass of filtered water after breakfast once a day, eventually working up to twice a day, after breakfast and after dinner. If you are new to taking fiber, start low and go slow, such as one-fourth teaspoon after breakfast. If no gas or bloating occurs, then slowly work your way up to a full or heaping teaspoon once or twice a day. (On a side note, you will want to rinse out your glass carefully, or the fiber will stick.)

For more insoluble fiber intake, I suggest nuts or nut butters, artichoke, cauliflower, broccoli, and other cruciferous veggies. For the veggies, it's the stems that have the most insoluble fiber, so be sure to eat those as well.

More to know about fiber

Constipation is terrible news for your gut. Besides causing pain, bloating, or even hemorrhoids, constipation decreases absorption of vitamins and minerals, allows the bad bacteria and fungi to multiply, increases leaky gut symptoms (including IBS, SIFO, and SIBO), and eventually affects your immune system.[7]

The answer is obviously to stop being constipated. One teaspoon of psyllium husk powder after breakfast and/or dinner will usually do the trick, as long as you are drinking sufficient amounts of water (at least eight cups per day).

Because fiber absorbs water, it increases the volume of your stools and helps move it all quickly through your GI tract.[8] Your body needs a quick process. Anything longer than the normal three-day cycle has the potential to cause you problems.

But here is something else interesting: fiber is similar to prebiotics in that it is beneficial not just for you but also for the good bacteria in your gut![9] Unlike proteins, carbs, or fats, fiber does not break down or get absorbed in your body. It is food for the good bacteria in your gut, especially in your colon. The fiber breaks down to feed your good bacteria, creating butyrate in the process, which is also a super fuel for your colon cells.[10]

Fiber is often called "roughage" or "bulk," but it is far more than that.

Your body desperately needs sufficient fiber every day, but most people are getting less than half of the fiber they need on a daily basis. Eventually, aim for 25–35 grams a day, and you can't go wrong. Add that to sufficient water intake, and you will often begin to see the magic of fiber after a week or two.

IT'S A FACT

Fiber and water do wonders for your gut. Be sure you drink enough water (at least eight cups per day), or the fiber may cause constipation.

Some of my patients have seen their cholesterol levels decrease 10–20 percent after a few months of psyllium fiber. Lower blood pressure levels and blood sugar levels are also common with my patients, which makes sense because soluble fiber supports healthy cholesterol and blood sugar levels. It also helps control appetite, which helps you lower your weight, thus lowering your blood pressure.

Other patients love it because it helps them lose weight. The fiber after breakfast and dinner makes them feel full longer, so they naturally eat less. But in their gut, the fiber makes the food pass through more quickly, which helps with proper absorption, lowers sugar levels, and fuels good gut bacteria growth, all of which helps with their metabolism. Fiber at night also helps reduce or stop late-night snacking.

We all need fiber, but if you suffer from SIFO, SIBO, or IBD, then fiber may cause bloating and gas. If you have colitis or Crohn's, fiber may cause a flare-up. What is the answer? Some doctors recommend avoiding fiber altogether until the patient's ailment, such as SIBO, is under control.

It is up to you, but I tell my patients to start low and go slow. Psyllium husk powder is usually soothing to the gut and brings with it many intrinsic healing properties, regardless of your symptoms or disease. Start with just one-quarter teaspoon of psyllium husk powder after breakfast and after a few days after dinner also. Every week increase it by one-quarter teaspoon until you reach one teaspoon or one heaping teaspoon twice a day. Your gut needs the many benefits of fiber, but if it takes you a while to get there, that is fine.

Fiber is one of those necessities for your gut health. Thankfully it is easy to come by.

Gut Power Tool 2: Probiotics

The second gut power tool is probiotics. Naturally, you may be wondering what probiotics are and what makes them so important for gut health. Good questions!

Probiotics are living organisms that improve the health of your gut, specifically the good bacteria in your gut biome. Here is a more technical definition if you prefer:

> Probiotics are "live microorganisms which when administered in adequate amounts confer a health benefit on the host."[11]

Like fiber, the focus of probiotics is not on you but on helping your gut be happy and healthy. Which, as you know, makes you happy in return! You can take probiotics as supplements in liquid, pill, or powder form, but probiotics are also found in many different foods and side dishes, such as these:

- kefir—a fermented milk (goat milk or coconut kefir preferred)
- kimchi—a spicy, fermented Korean dish
- kombucha—a tea made with sugar that is fermented by bacteria and yeast
- miso—a fermented Japanese soybean paste
- natto—fermented Japanese soybean product
- pickles—fermented and salty cucumbers
- sauerkraut—a fermented cabbage
- select cheeses—Gouda, mozzarella, cheddar, cottage (feta cheese preferred)
- tempeh—a fermented soybean patty
- traditional buttermilk—fermented dairy drink (goat milk buttermilk preferred)

- yogurt—with active or live cultures (goat milk or coconut yogurt preferred)[12]

How do these fit with your efforts to heal your gut? Though soybeans may be GMO or have lectins, eating probiotic-rich soybean-based foods to get the probiotics you need is probably not going to cause your gut too much distress because the fermenting process breaks down most of the lectins. If you are lactose intolerant or want to cut back on the small amount of milk sugar and A1 beta-casein in milk products (yogurt, kefir, and cheeses), choose probiotic-rich foods that have no milk, such as coconut kefir or coconut yogurt. Either way, you can choose from plenty of options that are full of probiotics and extremely healthy for your gut wall.

As of right now, five main probiotic species are well studied. Four of them are found in the food list you just read, and one of them is found in your birth mother. These five probiotics are as follows:

- *Lactobacillus plantarum*—found in many fresh or fermented veggies (i.e., kimchi, sauerkraut, pickles, brined olives)
- *Lactobacillus acidophilus*—found in fermented dairy options, such as yogurt and kefir (use caution with dairy, unless it is goat milk, coconut milk, or A2 milk kefir and yogurt)
- *Lactobacillus brevis*—found in sauerkraut and pickles
- *Bifidobacterium lactis*—found in fermented milk products, like yogurt and kefir (choose goat, coconut, or A2 milk products)
- *Bifidobacterium longum*—found in human mothers; babies get it when born naturally, especially when breastfed; also found in probiotic supplements[13]

There are thousands of different species of bacteria in the world and in your gut—many of them good and beneficial. This is a new frontier, one that is expanding and bringing more significant healing to our bodies as we learn more.

Probiotics have a relatively short shelf life in your gut. They are highly effective, but over time they will mostly disappear. That is why continued use of probiotics is necessary and effective.[14]

Some specialists are already using probiotics to treat ailments and diseases. For example, Dr. Michael Ruscio recommends these probiotics for the following conditions:

- celiac disease: lactobacilli and bifidobacteria
- IBD: lactobacilli and bifidobacteria, *Saccharomyces boulardii*, and *E. coli* Nissle 1917
- IBS/SIBO: lactobacilli and bifidobacteria
- mood/fatigue: lactobacilli and bifidobacteria
- weight loss: *Lactobacillus gasseri*[15]

In the very near future, I fully expect to see huge medical advances with probiotics. (See appendix B for a list of the most common probiotics that are in current use.)

Using probiotics to help your gut

One way to think of what probiotics do in your gut is to think of it this way:

1. Probiotics crowd out the bad bacteria and stop them from colonizing.

2. This minimizes ongoing damage to your gut while increasing the number of good bacteria.

3. The good bacteria then have room to grow and multiply, bringing healing to your gut and body.

That is the big picture of how probiotics go to work in your gut. Here is a quick, more specific list of what probiotics do for you at many different levels within your GI tract:

- absorb nutrients better[16]
- balance your gut bacteria[17]
- boost your immune system[18]
- fight infections[19]
- help your body digest protein[20]
- reduce inflammation[21]
- reduce your gut permeability[22]
- strengthen your gut lining[23]

But probiotics are something that you continually need to eat or take as supplements. One glass of goat milk kefir or one helping of sauerkraut is good for your gut, but just like with fiber, you need a daily intake of probiotics for your gut health. (See appendix D for powerful probiotics that I recommend to many of my patients.) I usually put my patients on at least one to two probiotic capsules a day and sometimes more. Sometimes I give them two to four different types of probiotics, depending on the severity of the dysbiosis and leaky gut. Occasionally, I will treat them with probiotic enemas.

IT'S A FACT

Probiotics are quick. Usually, in less than a week, your gut bacteria will have changed for the better.

As you work to daily include probiotics in your diet, keep in mind that it is good to shake things up a bit. Rotating probiotics after three to six months is recommended to keep your gut's microbiome diverse and healthy.[24] The more you do this naturally with the foods you eat, the happier your gut will be.

Some of my patients have been sick since childhood. Many of them use probiotic enemas to get massive amounts of probiotic organisms into their colon, which is where most of the good bacteria reside. Those enemas have worked wonders for many patients.

It's a bit more advanced, but if the need is there, you can try a probiotic enema. You can find many options online, but one simple routine involves an enema bag and a small amount of probiotic powder (the equivalent of six or more opened probiotic capsules) mixed well into filtered water. Make sure that your probiotic includes mainly bifidobacteria since these are the main bacteria in the colon. Follow the instructions that come with the enema bag. Do this after a morning bowel movement, and repeat one to three times a week for three to six weeks if needed. Attempt to retain the enema for twenty to thirty minutes if possible.

These probiotics help repair the gut lining, which immediately decreases inflammation. When the inflammation subsides, the symptoms usually disappear. This also typically helps to reduce every related risk of disease.

For most people, eating foods with probiotics or taking probiotic supplements is more than sufficient. Enemas are never fun, but if someone is really sick or has severe problems, the enema approach for getting high doses of probiotics into the system is a great option and is very beneficial. Many of my patients swear by this.

Further benefits of probiotics

With some specific symptoms or sicknesses, I recommend probiotics immediately. Other doctors have also found that probiotics help with such conditions as these:

- acne
- antibiotic-associated diarrhea (AAD)
- bacterial vaginosis (BV)
- dysbiosis
- infectious diarrhea
- IBD
- IBS
- leaky gut
- sinus infections
- traveler's diarrhea
- urinary tract infections (UTIs)
- yeast infections[25]

Probiotics stop, kill, or limit bad bacteria and bacterial growth while strengthening your intestinal wall and improving your immune system.[26] Those are great benefits!

Yes, probiotics mean using good bacteria against bad bacteria, but it works and has worked well for generations. Fermented milk products are thousands of years old, and interestingly enough, we are still learning just how beneficial these microscopic probiotics are.

Back in 1917, doctors wondered why one particular World War I soldier in the Balkans did not get severe diarrhea or any other intestinal disease like the rest of his comrades, many of whom died. Curious, researchers tested some of his stool samples and found a type of bacteria in his gut that the other soldiers did not have. A scientist named Alfred Nissle then bred that bacteria and packaged it into pills, and pills with that bacteria are still being produced to this day! More than one hundred years later, people are using that probiotic (named *E. coli* Nissle 1917) to help with their gut issues.[27]

But that is not all:

- Probiotics are used to fight depression.[28]
- Probiotics (called psychobiotics) are being used to improve and support mental health.[29]
- Probiotics (*Lactobacillus brevis* and *plantarum*, in particular) are used to increase BDNF, a brain-growth hormone.[30]
- Probiotics are used to improve your immune system.[31]
- Probiotics are used to reduce LPS in your body.[32]

If you are thinking, "What about probiotics and weight loss?" you are right on target. Dr. Steven Gundry clearly states: "The organisms in your intestines control how skinny or fat you will be."[33] The bacteria in your gut play a huge role in weight loss and weight gain.

IT'S A FACT

Chew your food well (twenty to thirty times per bite). Unchewed food benefits the bad bacteria in your gut by not being well absorbed and becoming their food.[34]

Is there a probiotic pill you can take that will make you lose weight? No, that has not yet been invented, though tests have been done that make that prospect look promising. But yes, much of the weight loss battle is waged in the gut.[35]

Even if a magic weight-loss pill existed, it would basically stop, kill, or limit bad bacteria, just like we can already do with the probiotic foods and supplements readily available. Proper food intake, exercise, and lifestyle choices would naturally be a part of the equation.

In 2014, researchers at the University of Toronto concluded, based on examining probiotic research up to that point, that "probiotics can be recommended for prevention of diseases that are associated to altered intestinal ecology."[36] Pretty much, that means probiotics are good, beneficial, and healthy for everything in your body and every disease that is connected in any way to your gut, which is practically everything!

GUT POWER TOOL 3: PREBIOTICS

The third gut power tool is prebiotics. Like probiotics, prebiotics are incredibly beneficial to your gut's microbiome and your entire GI tract. While probiotics are living organisms, prebiotics are more like insoluble fiber—undigestible and existing solely to serve your gut bacteria.

Here is a more extended definition: "Prebiotic fiber is a non-digestible part of foods...[that] goes through the small intestine undigested and is fermented when it reaches the large colon."[37] The fermenting action feeds the good bacteria in your colon.

Though prebiotics can be in supplement form, the most common way to get prebiotics is through the foods we eat. Many prebiotics are out there. Here are just a few of them:

- apples—better raw (best to avoid)
- asparagus—good cooked or raw
- bananas—the greener the better
- barley—a common cereal grain (best to avoid)
- burdock root—a common Japanese root
- chicory root—a coffee-like flavored root
- cocoa—a great flavoring or ingredient

- dandelion greens—great in salads
- flaxseeds—a healthy topping to many foods
- garlic—good for flavoring foods
- Jerusalem artichoke—great cooked or raw
- jicama root—good cooked or raw
- konjac root—also known as elephant yam, a tuber
- leeks—like onions, good raw or cooked
- oats—good cooked or raw (best to avoid)
- onions—good cooked or raw
- seaweed—common with many Asian dishes
- wheat bran—part of the whole wheat grain (best to avoid)
- yacon root—like a sweet potato[38]

Even more common foods with prebiotics include these:

- carrots
- coconut meat and milk (low fat)
- corn (best to avoid)
- pears (best to avoid)
- radishes
- tomatoes (best to avoid)[39]

Just as it was with fiber and probiotics, not every prebiotic is recommendable if you are working to restore your gut health. For starters, stay away from wheat bran, as that is super high in gluten. For a season, it would be advisable to steer clear of grains and legumes because of lectin content. Lastly, since you are keeping your sugars low, apples, pears, and ripe bananas should be avoided for the time being. Green bananas, however, have an extra benefit that we will soon discuss (gut power tool 5).

Using prebiotics to help your gut

To have a healthy gut, you must eventually feed your gut what it needs once the bloating and gas have been contained. That means prebiotics because prebiotics feed the good bacteria, and the good bacteria then can multiply and benefit your whole body.[40]

IT'S A FACT

Prebiotics must

- » *be nondigestible, which means they go through the stomach and small intestine without being broken down,*
- » *be fermented or metabolized by intestinal bacteria, and*
- » *give you health benefits.*[41]

Remember from the first chapter that there are two primary types of microbes in our gut—Firmicutes and Bacteroidetes—and how excessive Firmicutes make us fat while Bacteroidetes help us stay lean. Well, the prebiotic fibers in the many prebiotic foods actually feed, help, strengthen, and grow these same Bacteroidetes![42]

IT'S A FACT

"Prebiotics are specialized plant fibers. They . . . stimulate the growth of healthy bacteria in your gut."[43]

We cannot eliminate Firmicutes from our guts, as they are necessary for the health of the GI tract. When they overpopulate beyond the Bacteroidetes population, that's when we usually get fat. But when the Bacteroidetes are in control and dominate, we typically lose weight and get thinner. Consuming a diet high in sugar, carbs, and starches and low in fiber favors the growth of Firmicutes and more weight gain. However, a Healthy Gut Zone diet low in sugar, carbs, and starches and high in fiber and prebiotics favors the Bacteroidetes and helps with weight loss.

Prebiotics also produce butyrate, which I consider to be one of the most important benefits for your gut. That is because butyrate is a short-chain fatty acid (SFCA) and is fuel to the cells in your colon. Butyrate also has anti-inflammatory properties.[44] Decreasing inflammation in and of itself is a life changer for many people!

Because butyrate fuels your colon cells, it is praised for supporting your immune system and protecting against certain diseases of the digestive tract.[45] The more butyrate your gut has, the better off you will be.

Prebiotics also do the following:

- give you energy
- help with weight loss
- increase mineral (i.e., magnesium, calcium) absorption
- reverse common adverse effects of stomach acid blockers
- strengthen the probiotics already in your gut
- suppress hunger[46]

With my patients, I tell them to eventually aim for 12 grams of pre-biotics per day once gas and bloating have resolved. How much is that? If you are getting the fiber and probiotics your body needs, then adding about a handful of prebiotic foods to your daily diet should be sufficient. Use as many naturally prebiotic-rich vegetables in your salads or cooked meals as you want. The more it becomes a habit, the better.

IT'S A FACT

Despite what some people may say, sugar is not a prebiotic.

The only warning I have about prebiotics is for anyone who has been diagnosed with SIBO, SIFO, or IBD (Crohn's or ulcerative colitis). Prebiotics, though healthy, may cause more bloating and gas. If this occurs, stop taking any prebiotic supplements. You may be able to build up your prebiotic intake with natural foods slowly. Start low and go slow. Because your gut is getting healthier by the work you are doing to restore your gut, most likely the bloating and gas will decrease over time, and you will be able to enjoy prebiotics without bloating and gas.

GUT POWER TOOL 4: POLYPHENOLS

The fourth gut power tool has a strange name: polyphenols. You have eaten them before. In fact, you probably love them! But first, you are probably wondering what these polyphenols are and what makes them so important for your gut.

Polyphenols are antioxidant phytonutrients found in plants that do your body good! That's the best way to look at it. And more than eight thousand different polyphenols are out there![47]

A few of the most common sources of these healthy polyphenols include the following:

- berries (blueberries, raspberries, blackberries)
- black tea
- coffee
- dark chocolate (72 percent or more)
- green tea
- olive oils and olives (especially high-phenolic olive oil and oleocanthal)

Consuming these is certainly not going to be a problem! Here is a more detailed picture of where you can find polyphenols:

- fruits—apples, apricots, black elderberries, blackberries, black currants, blueberries, cherries, cranberries, grapefruit juice, grapes, oranges, peaches, plums, pomegranate juice, raspberries, strawberries (Modest amounts of berries—up to one-quarter or one-half cup a day—are fine, but most of the other fruits are too high in sugar.)
- vegetables—asparagus, black and green olives, broccoli, carrots, globe artichoke heads, onions, shallots, spinach (These foods are gut friendly.)
- whole grains—whole-grain oat, rye, and wheat flours (Avoid these foods.)

- nuts, seeds, legumes—almonds, black beans, chestnuts, flax-seeds, hazelnuts, pecans, roasted soybeans, walnuts, white beans (Nuts and flaxseeds are gut friendly.)
- beverages—coffee, tea, red wine (Coffee and tea are gut friendly, but avoid red wine for now.)
- fats—low-sugar dark chocolate, sesame seed oil, extra-virgin olive oil (Dark chocolate and olive oil are very gut friendly, but avoid sesame seed oil.)
- spices and seasonings—capers, celery seed, cinnamon, cloves, cocoa powder, cumin, curry powder, dried basil, dried ginger, dried oregano, dried peppermint, dried rosemary, dried sage, dried spearmint, dried thyme, saffron, soy sauce, star anise (Avoid soy sauce, and use caution with peppermint and spearmint for those with reflux.)[48]

There are also quite a few polyphenol supplements to choose from, such as these:

- grapeseed extract (supplement)
- green tea extract (supplement)
- pine bark extract (supplement)[49]

As with fiber, prebiotics, and probiotics, not every source of polyphenols is recommendable if you are working to restore your gut health. Staying low sugar/low fructose means avoiding all or most fruits and all fruit juices. Avoid grains and beans (because of lectins), but most nuts, spices, and seasonings are fine. Low-sugar dark chocolate (72 percent or greater) is an excellent source of polyphenols.

IT'S A FACT

Two squares of low-sugar dark chocolate (72 percent or higher) per day are a great source of polyphenols. I recommend eating them after dinner unless one has acid reflux.

Some of the many benefits of polyphenols

The fact that polyphenols contain antioxidants is an immediate good sign. Much is known about the power of antioxidants and how they clear free radicals out of your body. These free radicals increase inflammation in your body, and that leads directly to an increased risk of disease.[50]

To put it plainly, purposefully adding polyphenols to your diet will benefit you in many ways, including these:

- helping heal the gut[51]
- helping prevent long-term complications from diabetes[52]
- helping you lose weight by inhibiting fat cell development[53]
- improving bone metabolism, thereby reducing your risk of osteoporosis[54]
- improving the function of the endothelial cells in your arteries[55]
- lowering blood pressure[56]
- making you feel good[57]
- promoting brain health and cognitive function[58]
- protecting against dementia[59]
- reducing inflammation[60]
- reducing the effects of aging[61]
- reducing the risk of many cancers[62]
- relieving stress[63]

I have found polyphenols to be an extra boost to the proper F/B (Firmicute/Bacteroidetes) ratio that you want in your body.[64] Extra-virgin olive oil is, for me, the primary source of polyphenols as it makes the perfect salad dressing and can be drizzled over most cooked foods and added to soups.

Polyphenols are great for you, and you cannot get too much of them. The more, the better. I suggest trying to make it a daily habit to consume as many different polyphenols as you can, especially from high-phenolic extra-virgin olive oil (usually from Greek varieties), dark chocolate, and organic coffees.

GUT POWER TOOL 5: RESISTANT STARCHES

The fifth and final gut power tool is resistant starches. I define them as carbohydrates that are not digested (they resist it) until they reach the colon, where they ferment and feed the good bacteria in the gut.

Not every carb is a resistant starch. In fact, decreasing your carb intake to lower sugars is a necessary part of giving your gut time to heal. The bad bacteria thrive in a sugar-rich environment, while the good bacteria need a low-sugar environment to thrive.

IT'S A FACT

Oleocanthal is one of the most potent phenolic compounds or polyphenols in extra-virgin olive oil. It has anti-inflammatory activity, is anticarcinogenic, and prevents plaque formation in arteries.[65]

So, where do you find these resistant starches? Familiar food sources of resistant starches include these:

- beans, peas, and lentils (not gut friendly)
- corn, oats, barley, and rice (not gut friendly)
- green bananas (not fully ripened; gut friendly)
- green mangos (not fully ripened; gut friendly)
- green papaya (not fully ripened; gut friendly)
- green plantains (gut friendly)
- sweet potatoes (gut friendly)
- yams (gut friendly)

You are no doubt thinking (as with the lists of options for fiber, probiotics, prebiotics, and polyphenols) that not every option for resistant starches is going to be the right choice while you are trying to restore your gut health. That is true.

Resistant starches ferment in your colon, producing butyrate, which feeds the cells in the colon as well as the good bacteria.

Though beans, peas, and lentils have lectins, if you use a pressure cooker (cooking for at least seven and a half minutes, after soaking for twenty-four hours), the lectin content will usually be low enough not to stress your gut. For the first month or two, however, you should avoid beans, peas, and lentils while you are focusing on restoring your gut, and then follow the instructions for soaking and properly cooking them. Corn, oats, barley, and rice have a lot of carbs and lectins. I would avoid them for now as well.

As for the fruits, when the fruit is fully ripened, both the sugar/fructose content and lectin content are high. Eating the green fruit bypasses the sugar/fructose and lectins and provides you with a great source of resistant starches.

These fruits are good for your gut, but only when they are green. Sliced in bite-size pieces, they are a great topping on salads. That is always my recommendation for getting these resistant starches into a daily diet routine.

As with prebiotics, resistant starches produce butyrate, an incredibly valuable benefit. In fueling the cells in your gut, it decreases inflammation and helps feed the beneficial bacteria.[66]

Flours from green bananas and plantains are also available. They are great for cooking or baking, and the resistance starches feed the good bacteria in your gut.

Resistant starches are beneficial for your good gut bacteria. Work them into your diet. I buy green bananas and enjoy eating them, but when they turn yellow, I give them to my grandchildren. Start low and go slow to avoid bloating and gas.

CHAPTER ELEVEN

THE HEALTHY GUT ZONE DIET

HOW MANY PATIENTS who have come through my doors would have seen immediate relief of their symptoms or diseases had they jumped into the Healthy Gut Zone diet? The answer is thousands upon thousands!

Naturally, though many of them needed to take action, not all of them did. But I will say this: every patient I have had who took action to improve his or her gut health always had multiple health benefits come as a direct result. As I've tried to help you understand throughout this book, when you heal your gut, your entire body wins! And a happy gut is the foundation for a healthy body!

Now, you know I am not promising that every disease, sickness, ailment, or symptom will go away by following the Healthy Gut Zone diet. However, I have seen so much good happen with my patients, so many healthy prognoses after seemingly dead-end reports from doctors, that I encourage everyone to at least try it. What harm can it do to focus on your gut's health?

One of my recent patients was an eighty-year-old woman with kidney failure. How is that for a serious condition? She was on kidney dialysis, but within six months of starting the Healthy Gut Zone diet, she no longer had to go in for dialysis, and her doctors couldn't believe it. Her creatinine dropped from 2.6 to 1.6 in just a few months and stayed there.

Now, not everyone is faced with extreme health challenges like she was, but the simple act of getting her gut healthy again had amazing side effects on everything else in her body. She said she would stay on the Healthy Gut Zone diet for the rest of her life. The last time we spoke, she expressed her thanks at being healthy. Young or old, that is what everyone wants.

Patients with serious diseases, autoimmune diseases, and neurode-generative diseases (Alzheimer's, Parkinson's disease, and dementia) will need to stay on the Healthy Gut Zone diet and avoid most lectins. But the majority of patients with gut issues will eventually be able to eat most foods, as long as they limit or avoid sugar and wheat and rotate every three to four days any foods that may inflame their gut.

With that said, it is crucial to understand what is at the core of the Healthy Gut Zone diet. Here it is in straightforward terms:

1. **Feed the good.** The Healthy Gut Zone diet feeds the good bacteria in your gut the things that they need (i.e., probiotics, prebiotics, polyphenols, fiber, and resistant starches).

2. **Starve the bad.** The Healthy Gut Zone diet avoids, minimizes, or eliminates sugars, most starches and carbs, saturated fats, and foods that cause pain, inflammation, leaky gut, bloating, or irritation.

3. **Take time out.** The Healthy Gut Zone diet gives your gut time to catch its breath and heal itself.

That is all your GI tract needs. Your body is amazing in its ability to heal and recharge itself. And because the entire body is connected to the gut, we must get your gut healthy first. Everything else will follow.

With the Healthy Gut Zone diet, all three pieces (feed the gut, starve the bad, take time out) come together at the same time. The 1-2-3 tandem action is required by the gut, and it makes the whole process that much easier to implement.

FEEDING THE GOOD

With the gut, the underlying foundation is always that of making it healthy again. When the gut is healthy, you are usually happy. That is always the focus, no matter what.

"Feeding the good" means feeding the good bacteria in your gut what they need to be happy, healthy, and effective. You will be looking at food in that light, which means you will want to eat gut-friendly foods, such as the following.

Salads and vegetables

You want about one-half to two-thirds of each lunch and dinner to be raw or cooked veggies. See the list in appendix A.

The core or base of the Healthy Gut Zone diet is the veggies because that is what your gut needs the most. Thankfully there are endless recipe options, ways to prepare salads, soups, vegetables, and toppings. This diet also brings in healthy gut-friendly food options from different countries from around the world.

IT'S A FACT

Sugar and carbs grow yeast and bad bacteria in your gut. Those need to be avoided or minimized.

For lunch almost every day, I have a large salad with lots of veggies and a small amount of grilled chicken breast with grilled onions and a lot of high-phenolic extra-virgin olive oil (about four tablespoons). I don't put vinegar on it since vinegar decreases many of the polyphenols. But it is so tasty, and my wife and I have this almost every day. When your gut environment shifts from mostly Firmicutes to Bacteroidetes, your cravings usually shift from sugars, carbs, and starches to healthy foods. Now I actually crave salads with high-phenolic olive oil.

Proteins

You need protein from a variety of sources with almost every meal or snack. About one-fourth to one-third of each lunch and dinner should be protein. See appendix A for some of the many options for protein.

Everything else

In addition to the veggies and proteins are the fruits, fats, flours, resistant starches, and other things that accompany the Healthy Gut Zone diet. It's everything else that goes along with your veggies and proteins. These are important and healthy additions. (See appendix A.)

As you know, veggies are the base of the Healthy Gut Zone diet. Protein is a side but vitally important. Everything else is a complementary but necessary addition to the Healthy Gut Zone diet. All combined, your gut bacteria thrive on this mix of ingredients.

STARVING THE BAD

As you focus on consuming veggies, proteins, beverages, fermented foods, and other foods that support the growth of good gut bacteria, you simultaneously starve the bad bacteria. This is the other half of the equation, and it simply means that you avoid, minimize, or eliminate foods that cause pain, inflammation, leaky gut, bloating, or irritation.

If it hurts your gut, you don't eat it.

This concept of feeding the good and starving the bad is what your gut wants and needs. It is the perfect recipe for healing the GI tract.

How do you know what to avoid, minimize, or eliminate? The answer is in what you already know. You remember the seven causes of a leaky gut (increased intestinal permeability):

1. antibiotics

2. NSAIDs

3. acid-blocking meds

4. GMO foods

5. chlorine in drinking water

6. pesticides

7. intestinal infections

Starving the bad means not putting any more of items 1–6 into your body if you can help it. The biggest hurdle for many will be the fact that they are taking medications (items 1–3), whether doctor prescribed or over the counter. Abruptly stopping may not be advisable, and you may need to wean off meds such as antibiotics, acid blockers, NSAIDs, and aspirin under your doctor's care or under the care of a functional medicine doctor, but your gut needs a break.

IT'S A FACT

Too much saturated fat is not good for your gut. Foods high in saturated fat include butter, cream, cheese, coconut oil, fatty meats, lard, and palm oil.

DR. COLBERT'S HEALTHY GUT ZONE

So what should you do? I don't recommend stopping medications right away. Focus on healing the gut and let the body respond. The end goal is to add nothing to your gut that hurts it in any way. If it takes a few weeks before you can do that, then so be it. But the sooner, the better.

Most of the problems in the gut come from the seven causes of a leaky gut and the ten common enemies of the gut, which are mainly foods, including gluten. Though quitting something harmful for your gut will be a wise move, it is also essential to plant the good bacteria in your gut.

When the good bacteria are in control of your gut and the gut wall has healed, that is when the inflammation usually subsides. Many times, symptoms disappear, food sensitivities decrease, and sicknesses, even diseases, usually fade away. The psyllium husk powder also feeds the good bacteria and acts similar to a broom, sweeping out the bad bacteria and yeast.

To get to that point, starving the bad is required. These first seven common enemies must first be removed from your daily diet:

1. gluten

2. high-sugar, high-carb, high-processed foods

3. dairy

4. lectins

5. artificial sweeteners

6. emulsifiers

7. saturated fats

The shift away from these common enemies of the gut is more dramatic for some people than others, but it needs to happen nonetheless. The quicker, the better, but if it takes you a while, that is fine as well. When it comes to these first seven enemies of your gut, plan your escape this way:

Go *less*,
then go *low*, and
finally, go *none* at all.

For example, going gluten-free or lectin-free or sugar-free will not be a simple flip of a switch. It will take time to replace one food with another. Relax; don't put unnecessary pressure on yourself. Some changes may be immediate (e.g., not using artificial sweeteners), but others may take a little longer (e.g., going without dairy).

What is most important is that you are making lifelong habits of starving the bad bacteria while feeding the good bacteria. This is an ideal lifestyle, and your gut will be happy!

TAKING A TIME OUT

Looking at the big picture of your overall health and lifestyle going forward, you recognize that the change may need to be gradual. But you do need to start somewhere. There needs to be a break with the past and a rollout of the new. This is why the new year is such a popular time to try to make healthy changes. If you can't start at the beginning of a new year, I suggest that you embark on the Healthy Gut Zone diet as one season ends and another one begins.

When you begin, give yourself the expectation that you are jumping in completely and doing this for at least eight to twelve weeks (two to three months). You can do anything for just eight to twelve weeks, right? Naturally your body may love it so much that you wish to continue, but it is important that you mentally assign a window of time for your Healthy Gut Zone diet.

Usually the gut begins to heal within one to four weeks. I've had some patients feel the benefits immediately, but most start to feel the effects about four to seven days into it. That means symptoms often begin to fade away around the end of your first week!

While you are busy starving the bad bacteria and feeding the good bacteria, you will also be busy creating new habits that will further benefit your gut. Five complementary habits go in perfect tandem with the food-eating/food-avoiding habits you have already started. You already know these habits:

- Psyllium husk fiber—Take fiber (one-quarter to one teaspoon) one to two times daily, after breakfast and dinner, in four to eight ounces of water. (See appendix D.)

- Probiotics—Take one to four probiotics per day or eat probiotic-rich foods. (Add supplements if needed. See appendix D.)

- Prebiotics—Take 12 grams of prebiotic supplements (add prebiotic-rich foods if you can) a day. Start with much less if you have bloating or gas. Use caution if you have SIBO, SIFO, Crohn's disease, or ulcerative colitis; hold off, or start low and go slow.

- Polyphenols—Add as many polyphenols to your daily routine as you can.

- Resistant starches—These add options to your diet as they feed your good gut bacteria. Use caution if you have bloating, gas, SIBO, SIFO, Crohn's disease, or ulcerative colitis; hold off, or start low and go slow.

IT'S A FACT

The Healthy Gut Zone diet schedule:

» *Phase One: give intense focus for eight to twelve weeks.*

» *Phase Two: expand food choices for two to three more months.*

» *Phase Three: live a gut-friendly lifestyle of ongoing good habits.*

After eight weeks, you can begin to add back into your diet certain foods that you might want to avoid completely at first. For example, I recommend that you stay off cucumbers, tomatoes, eggplant, and peppers during the initial part of your Healthy Gut Zone diet. This minimizes lectins. After a couple of months, by peeling and deseeding these vegetables, you may be able to eat them with only a slight increase in lectin exposure (since lectins are more concentrated in the seeds and skins).

With beans, which are excellent sources of protein, pressure-cooking them for seven and a half minutes or longer after twenty-four hours of soaking (discard the water they are soaked in) will break down and remove virtually all the lectins, making them safe to eat. But during the first one to two months of your Healthy Gut Zone diet, I would recommend not eating beans at all.

IT'S A FACT

Unless your gut is healthy, a weight-loss diet is only a temporary fix.

In addition to watching lectins, you always have to be aware of sugars (i.e., fructose in fruits), carbohydrates (i.e., in legumes), grains, saturated fats (i.e., in dairy products), and fatty cuts of meat. For your gut, while it is healing, the longer you can stay low sugar, low carb, and low saturated fats, the better. As for gluten, I recommend that most people pretty much stay off gluten, though an occasional small amount of food containing gluten will usually not hurt.

When you begin to slowly increase your food options, such as adding a new food each week, keep in mind that you will want to stay within the overall Healthy Gut Zone framework of starving the bad and feeding the good. That means continually avoiding the seven causes of a leaky gut and the first seven common enemies of your gut. You know what those are.

When you add dairy back, start with sheep or goat milk products or A2 dairy. For example, I enjoy some feta cheese in my Greek salad. Choose low-fat, low-sugar goat milk that is fermented, such as goat milk yogurt or kefir. Eventually you can add small amounts of A2 milk or two to four ounces of low-fat cheese and rotate it every three to four days.

Usually within three months you can add back in foods you love, such as Indian basmati white rice (limit to one-half cup per serving) or potatoes without the skin (where the most lectins are found). Rotate this food as well as other high-lectin foods every two to four days, and avoid any high-lectin food that causes abdominal pain, excessive bloating, gas, or other symptoms of leaky gut. Rotating foods that are inflammatory for you or high in lectins is a great way to still enjoy them yet limit them so they are less likely to harm the gut. But do not add in sugar foods, gluten, GMO foods, or excessive foods high in saturated fats.

Stay with it. Most people will find that their gut is healed within three months.

THE HEALTHY GUT ZONE LIFESTYLE

This has always been about more than just a diet. It is about getting healthy and staying healthy, and that is the result of a lifestyle more than anything.

If any symptoms you eradicated from your life reoccur, then examine what you are eating. The old "normalness" of bloating, gas, diarrhea, nose running, brain fog, fatigue, achy joints, etc. became a thing of the past, and they should stay there.

You don't need inflammation of any sort. So pay attention to your gut and adjust as needed. After several months on the Healthy Gut Zone diet, most people find that their food sensitivities noticeably faded away. Are those sensitivities gone forever? Perhaps, but maybe not. A healthy gut can handle the occasional food that isn't Healthy Gut Zone friendly, but it should remain occasional and not part of a daily routine. That is why rotating certain foods that used to irritate your gut every three to four days is so beneficial to your gut.

As I mentioned earlier, if you have an autoimmune disease, you may need to stay on the Healthy Gut Zone diet for a lot longer, and you may have to avoid most high-lectin foods and especially gluten. If it brings you the relief and health you want and need, I suggest that you make it your permanent lifestyle.

Many patients have told me that after they stopped having their symptoms, sickness, or disease, they intended to stay on the Healthy Gut Zone diet forever. It is a doable diet, a diet that always tries to make your gut happy.

And if your gut is happy, you are healthy. That is always the goal.

Children will need adequate starches for calories and growth in the form of Indian white basmati rice, which has much fewer lectins, and eventually pressure-cooked beans, peas, and lentils. Also, sweet potatoes, yams, carrots, millet bread, yucca, taro root, and jicama are all gut-friendly carbs. Cassava and cassava chips with lime are a tasty, gut-friendly carb. Also, cauliflower chips (lime flavor) are another good option.

CHAPTER TWELVE

A WEEK IN THE HEALTHY GUT ZONE

STAYING IN THE Healthy Gut Zone is the goal. Here is a week of recipes that can keep you there.

DAY 1

BREAKFAST

Organic coffee with 1 scoop MCT oil
½ to 1 teaspoon psyllium husk powder in 4 ounces of water

SMOOTHIE

8 ounces almond or low-fat, low-sugar coconut milk
2 tablespoons avocado oil
½ to 1 scoop egg white protein (if not sensitive to egg) or
    collagen protein
¼ cup frozen berries
Stevia

Blend first four ingredients. Sweeten to taste with stevia. Add ice if desired.

OR

HEALTHY GUT ZONE FLAPJACKS

2 eggs
½ cup green banana flour or sweet potato flour
Pinch of salt
Water
Pinch of cinnamon
Fresh blueberries or blackberries

Avocado oil
Grass-fed butter

Combine eggs, flour, salt, water, and cinnamon. Pour into a griddle or frying pan flip to brown both sides. Simmer berries in 2 tablespoons avocado oil under low heat. Top flapjacks with berries and a pat of grass-fed butter.

LUNCH

1 small sweet potato (may add Pyure stevia and cinnamon)

GRILLED CHICKEN SALAD

Large salad greens
Onions, chopped or sliced
Mushrooms, chopped or sliced
Celery, chopped or sliced
Fresh parsley
2–4 tablespoons extra-virgin olive oil (may add lemon juice and/or vinegar)
3–6 ounces boneless organic free-range chicken breast, grilled
Grilled onions

Toss salad greens with vegetables and parsley. Drizzle with olive oil, and top with grilled chicken and grilled onions.

DINNER

CURRY SOUP

Gut-friendly veggies of your choice (such as onions, carrots, celery, garlic, broccoli, mushrooms), diced or chopped
1 boneless organic free-range chicken breast, diced or shredded
1 tablespoon yellow curry powder
2 cups organic chicken stock
½ cup low-fat coconut milk
1 tablespoon freshly squeezed lime juice
4–6 tablespoons extra-virgin olive oil or avocado oil
Salt

In a stockpot, combine your choice of gut-friendly veggies with chicken breast, curry powder, chicken stock, coconut milk, and lime juice. Season with salt as desired. Simmer for 25 minutes on medium heat. After simmering and before serving, add olive oil or avocado oil. Serves 2.

DAY 2

BREAKFAST

Organic coffee with 1 scoop MCT oil
½ to 1 teaspoon psyllium husk powder in 4 ounces of water
2–3 organic pastured eggs, scrambled with onions, mushrooms, and garlic in avocado oil
½ avocado sliced
¼ cup berries

LUNCH

1 green banana

GRILLED SALMON SALAD

Romaine lettuce, chopped
Onions, chopped or sliced
Mushrooms, chopped or sliced
Carrots, chopped or sliced
Celery, chopped or sliced
2–4 tablespoons extra-virgin olive oil (may add lemon juice and/or vinegar)
3–6 ounces wild salmon, grilled

Toss romaine lettuce with vegetables. Drizzle with olive oil, and top with grilled salmon.

DINNER

TORTILLA-LESS CHICKEN SOUP

1 small onion, diced
1–2 teaspoons minced garlic

3 cups organic chicken stock

9–12 ounces boneless organic free-range chicken breast,
   boiled and shredded

1 tablespoon freshly squeezed lime juice

⅓ to ½ cup fresh cilantro leaves, chopped

1 avocado, sliced or cubed

½ to 1 cup mushrooms (if desired)

½ to 1 cup broccoli (if desired)

6–8 tablespoons extra-virgin olive oil

In a stockpot, combine first nine ingredients. Simmer 25 minutes on medium heat. After simmering and before serving, add olive oil. Serves 3.

DAY 3

BREAKFAST

Organic coffee with 1 scoop MCT oil

½ to 1 teaspoon psyllium husk powder in 4 ounces of water

MILLET BREAD FRENCH TOAST

2 large brown organic pastured eggs

1 teaspoon organic vanilla extract

½ teaspoon ground cinnamon

½ cup low-fat coconut milk

1 teaspoon Pyure granulated stevia

2 slices millet bread

Avocado oil

¼ cup berries (if desired)

Grass-fed butter (if desired)

Make a batter by whisking together eggs, vanilla extract, cinnamon, coconut milk, and stevia. Soak each slice of millet bread in batter. Cook in skillet using avocado oil under low heat. Add berries simmered in 2 tablespoons avocado oil and a pat of grass-fed butter as a topping if desired. Serves 2.

OR

CHOCOLATE SMOOTHIE

½ teaspoon dark sugar-free cocoa
½ teaspoon Pyure stevia
1 tablespoon almond butter
1 tablespoon avocado oil
1 scoop chocolate hydrolyzed collagen protein (See appendix D.)
8 ounces almond or low-fat, low-sugar coconut milk

Blend all ingredients. Add ice if desired.

LUNCH

SIMPLE TURKEY SALAD

Spinach
2–4 tablespoons olive oil (may add lemon juice and/or vinegar)
3–6 ounces turkey
Green mango and/or green papaya, sliced

Toss spinach with olive oil. Top with turkey, and add slices of green mango and/or green papaya.

DINNER

WILD SHRIMP GUMBO

8 ounces wild shrimp
2–3 cups organic chicken stock
½ cup onion, chopped
½ cup celery, chopped
2 garlic cloves, minced
½ cup fresh okra
Salt
Pepper
4–6 tablespoons extra-virgin olive oil

In a stockpot, combine first six ingredients. Add salt and pepper to taste. Simmer for 25–30 minutes. After simmering and before serving, add olive oil. Serves 2.

DAY 4

BREAKFAST

Organic coffee with 1 scoop MCT oil, ½ teaspoon dark
  cocoa powder, and stevia (if desired)
½ to 1 teaspoon psyllium husk powder in 4 ounces of water
Omelet cooked in avocado oil with onions, mushrooms, and
  garlic
½ avocado, sliced
¼ cup berries

LUNCH

1 green banana

CHICKEN SALAD

1 boneless organic free-range chicken breast
2 celery stalks
½ onion
Salt
Pepper
½ cup pecans
⅓ cup avocado oil mayonnaise
1 tablespoon fresh dill, chopped (if desired)
1 tablespoon Dijon mustard (if desired)
2 tablespoons extra-virgin olive oil or avocado oil
2 large romaine lettuce leaves

Boil chicken breast in water with celery stalks, onion, salt, and pepper for 20–25 minutes. Once cooked, chill chicken in refrigerator while making rest of salad.

Chop the cooked celery and onion into small pieces. Add pecans, mayonnaise, and, if desired, fresh dill and Dijon mustard. Season with salt and pepper to taste. Add shredded chicken and olive oil or avocado oil to rest of ingredients. Mix well.

Serve 1–2 scoops on large leaf of romaine lettuce. Serves 2.

Optional: You may make a sandwich using millet bread or breads in appendix A under starches. However, a low-carb diet works better for the first month.

DINNER

GRASS-FED BEEF SOUP

2–4 cups organic beef stock
Gut-friendly veggies of your choice (such as onions, carrots,
   mushrooms, and broccoli), diced or chopped
Garlic
8 ounces grass-fed, grass-finished lean filet mignon, grilled
   and diced
Salt
Pepper
4–6 tablespoons extra-virgin olive oil or avocado oil

In a stockpot, combine first four ingredients. Season with salt and pepper to taste. Simmer for 25 minutes or longer. After simmering and before serving, add olive oil or avocado oil. Serves 2.

DAY 5

BREAKFAST

Organic coffee with 1 scoop MCT oil, ½ teaspoon dark
   cocoa powder, and stevia (if desired)
½ to 1 teaspoon psyllium husk powder in 4 ounces of water
1 scoop chocolate or vanilla hydrolyzed collagen protein in 6
   ounces of water in a shaker bottle (See appendix D.)

LUNCH

TONGOL TUNA SALAD

1 can tongol tuna
2 celery stalks
½ onion
½ cup pecans
⅓ cup avocado oil mayonnaise
1 tablespoon fresh dill, chopped (if desired)
1 tablespoon Dijon mustard (if desired)

Salt

Pepper

2 tablespoons extra-virgin olive oil or avocado oil

Green mango, sliced

2 large romaine lettuce leaves

Open can of tongol tuna, and chill tuna in refrigerator while making rest of salad.

Chop celery and onion into small pieces. Add pecans, mayonnaise, and, if desired, fresh dill and Dijon mustard. Season with salt and pepper to taste. Add tuna and olive oil or avocado oil to rest of ingredients. Add slices of green mango. Mix well.

Serve 1–2 scoops on large leaf of romaine lettuce. Serves 2.

Optional: You may make a tuna sandwich using millet bread or breads listed under starches in appendix A.

DINNER

BONE BROTH SOUP

BONE BROTH:

Water

Boneless, skinless chicken OR grass-fed, grass-finished low-
fat beef or steak

Boil chicken or beef/steak for 20 minutes. Once cooled, remove meat and shred or cube it.

SOUP:

2 cups bone broth

Chicken or beef/steak from bone broth, shredded or cubed

½ cup onions, chopped

½ cup broccoli, chopped

½ cup celery, chopped

2 garlic cloves, minced

Salt

Pepper

4–6 tablespoons extra-virgin olive oil or avocado oil

In a stockpot, combine first six ingredients. Season with salt and pepper to taste. Simmer for 25 minutes. After simmering and before serving, add olive oil or avocado oil. Serves 2.

DAY 6

BREAKFAST

Organic coffee with 1 scoop MCT oil
½ to 1 teaspoon psyllium husk powder in 4 ounces of water

SMOOTHIE

8 ounces almond or low-fat, low-sugar coconut milk
2 tablespoons avocado oil
½ to 1 scoop egg white protein (if not sensitive to egg) or hydrolyzed collagen protein
¼ cup frozen berries
Stevia

Blend first four ingredients. Sweeten with stevia to taste. Add ice if desired.

LUNCH

GRILLED CHICKEN SALAD

Mixed salad greens
Onions, chopped or sliced
Mushrooms, chopped or sliced
Carrots, chopped or sliced
Celery, chopped or sliced
2–4 tablespoons extra-virgin olive oil (may add lemon juice and/or vinegar)
3–6 ounces boneless organic free-range chicken breast, grilled

Toss mixed greens with veggies. Drizzle with olive oil, and top with grilled chicken.

DINNER

1 small sweet potato (may add Pyure stevia and cinnamon)

KALE AND VEGGIE SALAD WITH CHICKEN

4 cups (packed) kale leaves, torn, with stems removed
½ cup large avocado, chopped
⅓ cup red onion
½ cup English cucumber, deseeded and chopped
Handful of pomegranate seeds
1 radish, thinly sliced
1 celery stalk, chopped
2–4 tablespoons extra-virgin olive oil
2 tablespoons freshly squeezed lime juice
¼ cup cilantro, diced (if desired)
3–6 ounces boneless organic free-range chicken, grilled

Toss together first ten ingredients. Top with grilled chicken.

DAY 7

BREAKFAST

Organic coffee with 1 scoop MCT oil
½ to 1 teaspoon psyllium husk powder in 4 ounces of water

CHOCOLATE SMOOTHIE

½ teaspoon dark sugar-free cocoa
½ teaspoon Pyure stevia
1 tablespoon almond butter
1 tablespoon avocado oil
1 scoop chocolate hydrolyzed collagen protein
8 ounces almond or low-fat, low-sugar coconut milk

Blend all ingredients. Add ice if desired.

LUNCH

SPICY GINGER SALAD WITH CHICKEN OR BEEF

> Cabbage (green, purple, or mixed), chopped or shredded
> Carrots, chopped or sliced
> Radishes, sliced
> Parsnips, chopped or sliced
> Onions, chopped or sliced
> Celery, chopped or sliced
> 2 tablespoons fresh ginger
> 2–4 tablespoons extra-virgin olive oil (may add lemon juice and/or vinegar)
> 3–6 ounces lean grass-fed, grass-finished beef OR boneless organic free-range chicken, grilled and cut in strips

Toss cabbage with other veggies. Grate or dice ginger over top. Drizzle with olive oil, and top with strips of grilled beef or chicken.

DINNER

CREAMY CARROT CHICKEN AND COCONUT SOUP

> 2–3 large carrots, finely chopped
> 14-ounce can low-fat coconut milk
> 1 onion, finely chopped
> 1 tablespoon curry powder
> 1 teaspoon fresh ginger, minced
> 2 cups organic vegetable or chicken broth
> 8 ounces boneless organic free-range chicken, boiled and shredded
> Salt
> Pepper
> 4–6 tablespoons extra-virgin olive oil or avocado oil

In a stockpot, combine first seven ingredients. Season with salt and pepper to taste. Simmer for 25 minutes. After simmering and before serving, add olive oil or avocado oil. Serves 2.

CONCLUSION

THE MORE WE learn about the gut and its connectedness to the brain, immune system, digestion, disease prevention, and overall health, the more you will hear others begin to champion the same message you've read in this book:

- *Feed* your gut.
- *Protect* your gut.
- *Heal* your gut.
- *Balance* your gut.

You will know what they are talking about, and it makes good sense because when your gut is happy, your body is healthy.

So whatever symptoms you or your family might face, the odds are incredibly high that they're connected to your gut. Literally, from head to toe, every part of your body is impacted by the health of your gut.

Thankfully, good gut health is within reach. It's doable.

My wish for you is that you find the relief, healing, and health that you are looking for. And because all healing begins in the gut, I am genuinely excited for you!

HEALING FOODS

PUT THESE FOODS at the top of your shopping list while on the Healthy Gut Zone diet.

Veggies: artichokes, arugula, asparagus, basil, beets, bok choy, broccoli, brussels sprouts, cabbage (Chinese, green, red), carrots, cauliflower, celery, chives, cilantro, cucumbers (if peeled and deseeded), garlic, greens (collard, dandelion, field, mustard), kale, kimchi, kohlrabi, lettuce (butter, romaine, green leaf, red leaf), mint, mushrooms, okra, olives, onions (all types), parsley, perilla, purslane, radishes, sauerkraut, scallions, seaweed, spinach, Swiss chard, tomatoes (if peeled and deseeded), watercress

Dairy: Avoid all dairy for one to three months. After that, use cheese (goat, sheep, feta), grass-fed butter, grass-fed ghee, goat milk kefir, goat milk yogurt, milk (goat or A2 milk rather than A1).

Meat: beef, bison, elk, lamb, moose, venison (all known to be or listed as grass-fed and grass-finished); chicken, duck, eggs, goose, pheasant, quail, turkey (all known to be or listed as organic and free-range, not fed soybeans); anchovies, bass, calamari, clams, crab, halibut, lobster, mussels, oysters, salmon, sardines, scallops, shrimp, tongol tuna (all known to be or listed as wild)

Nuts and seeds: almonds, Brazil nuts, chestnuts, coconut, flax-seeds, hazelnuts, macadamia, pecans, pine nuts, pistachio, psyllium, walnuts. Note that peanuts and cashews are not nuts but legumes.

Beverages: coffee; tea (black, green); filtered water, spring water, or sparkling water with lemon or lime wedge

Chocolate: low-sugar dark (72 percent or higher)

Fats: avocado, MCT, nut, and olive oils

Fermented foods: kimchi, pickles, sauerkraut

Flours: almond, arrowroot, cassava, coconut, green banana, plantain, sweet potato flour

Fruits: avocado and berries (blueberries, blackberries, raspberries, strawberries). These are the best due to their low sugar content.

Resistant starches: green banana, green mango, green papaya, jicama, parsnips, rutabaga, sweet potato, taro root, yams, yucca

Seasonings: anise, basil, capers, celery seed, cinnamon, cloves, cocoa powder, cumin, curry powder, ginger, oregano, peppermint, rosemary, saffron, sage, spearmint, thyme

Starches: flax bread, millet bread. Add Indian basmati white rice after avoiding for at least one month, sweet potatoes, yams, cassava, carrots, taro root, yucca, jicama, tortillas (from cassava, cassava and coconut, or almond by Siete brand), and bread made from almond, coconut, or cassava, such as Julian Bakery paleo bread.

Supplements: prebiotics, probiotics, psyllium husk powder, and, if needed, vitamin D_3, hydrolyzed collagen, L-glutamine, magnesium, omega-3 (See appendix D.)

Sweeteners: erythritol, Just Like Sugar (inulin), monk fruit sugar, stevia

APPENDIX B

COMMON PROBIOTICS

THIS IS A list of many of the well-researched, gut-friendly probiotics that are readily available in foods or supplements.

Lactobacillus acidophilus: helps decrease bad bacteria growth, helps maintain gut bacteria balance, helps reduce yeast infections[1]

Lactobacillus brevis: helps reduce LPS, strengthens gut wall, improves immune function[2]

Lactobacillus casei: helps heal infectious diarrhea[3]

Lactobacillus gasseri: helps treat *H. pylori*[4]

Lactobacillus plantarum: helps heal infectious diarrhea, helps decrease inflammation, helps maintain gut bacteria balance[5]

Lactobacillus rhamnosus: helps prevent diarrhea[6]

Lactobacillus salivarius: helps reduce gas[7]

Streptococcus thermophilus: helps digest lactose[8]

Bifidobacterium bifidum: is beneficial for the immune system[9]

Bifidobacterium infantis: helps with IBS[10]

Bifidobacterium longum: helps prevent diarrhea and constipation, helps improve lactose tolerance[11]

Bifidobacterium lactis: helps decrease bloating, strengthens gut wall, helps boost immunity[12]

Saccharomyces boulardii: helps heal infectious diarrhea[13]

FOODS THAT CONTAIN GLUTEN

LUTEN IS THE protein found in certain grains and most bread, pasta, bagels, pretzels, cereals, cakes, cookies, and processed foods. A 2019 Healthline article highlights the following foods that may or do contain gluten.[1] You'll want to avoid these foods while you're on the Healthy Gut Zone diet.

Grains with gluten:

- barley
- rye
- triticale
- wheat

Fruits and vegetables that may include gluten:

- canned—the sauce may contain gluten
- dried—may have added gluten ingredients
- frozen—flavoring and sauces may contain gluten
- prechopped—may be cross-contaminated with gluten

Proteins that may or do include gluten:

- breaded meats of any kind—contain gluten
- ground meats
- hot dogs, pepperoni, sausage, salami, bacon
- lunch meats/cold cuts
- microwavable TV dinners
- proteins with soy sauce—contains gluten[2]

- seitan—contains gluten
- vegetarian burgers

Dairy products that may or do include gluten:

- flavored milk and yogurt
- ice cream if additives have gluten
- malted milk drinks—contain gluten
- processed cheese products, like cheese sauces/spreads

Fats/oils that may include gluten:
- cooking sprays
- oils with added flavors/spices

Beverages that may or do include gluten:

- bccrs, alcs, and lagers—made from grains
- drinks with added flavorings
- premade smoothies
- wine coolers—contain gluten[3]

Spices, sauces, and condiments that may include gluten:

- barbecue sauce
- dry spices
- gravy and stuffing mixes
- ketchup and mustard
- malt vinegar—contains gluten[4]
- marinades
- mayonnaise
- pasta sauce
- relish and pickles
- rice vinegar
- salad dressing

- salsa
- stock and bouillon cubes
- teriyaki sauce—contains gluten[5]
- tomato sauce
- wheat-based soy sauce—contains gluten
- Worcestershire sauce

GUT-FRIENDLY SUPPLEMENTS

THE FOLLOWING SUPPLEMENTS are beneficial for your gut, gut health, GI tract, and entire body.

Divine Health supplements
Available at shop.drcolbert.com or by calling (407) 732-6952

- Fiber Zone: great-tasting psyllium husk powder with prebiotics (inulin); available flavors: berry or unflavored (contains soluble and insoluble fibers)
- Hydrolyzed Collagen: powder that helps repair a leaky gut; available flavors: vanilla, chocolate, or unflavored
- Green Supremefood: superfood drink with ten organic fermented veggies and no nightshades, with probiotics
- Red Supremefood contains nine organic fruits and is low-sugar and includes raspberry, blueberry, cranberry, acai, and pomegranate.
- MCT oil powder: adding one to two scoops a day to coffee (along with Pyure stevia) provides healthy fats that convert to ketones; contains prebiotics; available flavors: coconut, Dutch chocolate, French vanilla, hazelnut, unflavored
- Living Probiotic: a powerful probiotic to help restore a leaky gut; contains *Bifidobacterium breve*, *Bifidobacterium lactis*, and *Lactobacillus plantarum*. Available from trybeyond biotics.com

Dr. Colbert's office phone number: (407) 331-7007

Other recommended supplements

- Visbiome (for IBS, ulcerative colitis, and Crohn's disease) 112.5 billion CFU per capsule. www.visbiome.com
- Vitamin D_3 2000 IU
- Spore-based probiotics such as these can form spores and are highly resistant to stomach acid:
  - « MegaSporeBiotic by Microbiome Labs; available at https://microbiomelabs.com/home/products/megasporebiotic/
  - « BioSpora from Klaire Labs; available at https://klaire.com/k-bsp-12-biospora

If a patient has severe leaky gut and dysbiosis, I commonly place him or her on two or more types of probiotics such as Living Probiotic and BioSpora.

NOTES

INTRODUCTION

1. Robynne Chutkan, *The Microbiome Solution: A Radical New Way to Heal Your Body from the Inside Out* (New York: Avery, 2015), 3.

2. Cell Press, "Gut Microbes Signal to the Brain When They're Full," ScienceDaily, November 24, 2015, https://www.sciencedaily.com/releases/2015/11/151124143330.htm.

3. Siri Carpenter, "That Gut Feeling," *Monitor on Psychology* 43, no. 8 (September 2012): 50, https://www.apa.org/monitor/2012/09/gut-feeling.

4. John B. Furness, Wolfgang A. Kunze, and Nadine Clerc, "Nutrient Tasting and Signaling Mechanisms in the Gut. II. The Intestine as a Sensory Organ: Neural, Endocrine, and Immune Responses," *The American Journal of Physiology* 277, no. 5 (November 1999): G922–28, https://pubmed.ncbi.nlm.nih.gov/10564096/.

5. "The Central Role of the Gut," Danone Nutricia Research, accessed July 13, 2020, https://nutriciaresearch.com/gut-and-microbiology/the-central-role-of-the-gut/.

CHAPTER 1

1. "Strangest Diet," Guinness World Records, accessed July 18, 2020, https://www.guinnessworldrecords.com/world-records/67621-strangest-diet.

2. Emanuele Rinninella et al., "What Is the Healthy Gut Microbiota Composition? A Changing Ecosystem Across Age, Environment, Diet, and Diseases," *Microorganisms* 7, no. 1 (January 10, 2019): 14, https://www.ncbi.nlm.nih.gov/pmc/articles/PMC6351938/.

3. Chutkan, *The Microbiome Solution*, 14.

4. Rob Knight and Daniel McDonald, "Our Second Genome," *Imagine* (September–October 2013), https://cty.jhu.edu/imagine/docs/second-genome.pdf.

5. Giulia Enders, *Gut: The Inside Story of Our Body's Most Underrated Organ* (Vancouver, BC: Greystone, 2015), 161.

6. Enders, *Gut*, 148.

7. Sahil Khanna and Pritish K. Tosh, "A Clinician's Primer on the Role of the Microbiome in Human Health and Disease," *Mayo Clinic Proceedings* 89, no. 1 (January 2014): 107–14, https://www.mayoclinicproceedings.org/article/S0025-6196(13)00886-0/fulltext.

8. Rinninella et al., "What Is the Healthy Gut Microbiota Composition? A Changing Ecosystem Across Age, Environment, Diet, and Diseases."

9. David Perlmutter with Kristin Loberg, *Brain Maker: The Power of Gut Microbes to Heal and Protect Your Brain—for Life*, (New York: Little, Brown Spark, 2015), 31, https://www.amazon.com/Brain-Maker-Power-Microbes-Protect/dp/1478985550.

10. Enders, *Gut*, 162–63.

11. Amy Kraft, "C-Section Births Linked to Long-Term Child Health Problems," CBS News, June 11, 2015, https://www.cbsnews.com/news/c-section-cesarean-births-child-health-problems-asthma-obesity-diabetes/.

12. Shahrokh Amiri et al., "Pregnancy-Related Maternal Risk Factors of Attention-Deficit Hyperactivity Disorder: A Case-Control Study," *International Scholarly Research Notices*, 2012, https://www.hindawi.com/journals/isrn/2012/458064/.

13. Chutkan, *The Microbiome Solution*, 5.

14. Gaby Galvin, "Study: C-Section Tied to Higher Risk of Autism," *U.S. News and World Report*, August 28, 2019, https://www.usnews.com/news/health-news/articles/2019-08-28/c-section-tied-to-higher-risk-of-autism-adhd.

15. Evalotte Decker et al., "Cesarean Delivery Is Associated with Celiac Disease but Not Inflammatory Bowel Disease in Children," *Pediatrics* 125, no. 6 (June 2010): e1433–40, https://pediatrics.aappublications.org/content/125/6/e1433.

16. Kraft, "C-Section Births Linked to Long-Term Child Health Problems"; Perlmutter, *Brain Maker*, 36.

17. Niall McCarthy, "Which Countries Conduct the Most Cesarean Sections?" Statista, October 16, 2018, https://www.statista.com/chart/15787/caesarean-rates-by-country/; Conor Stewart, "Share of Childbirths Delivered by Cesarean Section in Europe in 2015, by Country," Statista, February 13, 2020, https://www.statista.com/statistics/953812/births-by-caesarean-section-in-europe/.

18. Stefani Lobionda et al., "The Role of Gut Microbiota in Intestinal Inflammation with Respect to Diet and Extrinsic Stressors," *Microorganisms* 7, no. 8 (August 2019): 271, https://www.ncbi.nlm.nih.gov/pmc/articles/PMC6722800/#B10-microorganisms-07-00271.

19. Lobionda et al., "The Role of Gut Microbiota in Intestinal Inflammation with Respect to Diet and Extrinsic Stressors."

20. Lobionda et al., "The Role of Gut Microbiota in Intestinal Inflammation with Respect to Diet and Extrinsic Stressors."

21. Yasmine Belkaid and Timothy Hand, "Role of the Microbiota in Immunity and Inflammation," *Cell* 157, no. 1 (March 27, 2014): 121–41, https://www.ncbi.nlm.nih.gov/pmc/articles/PMC4056765/.

22. University of Bern, "Gut Microbes Shape Our Antibodies Before We Are Infected by Pathogens," Medical Xpress, August 5, 2020, https://medicalxpress.com/news/2020-08-gut-microbes-antibodies-infected-pathogens.html.

23. Gerard Clarke et al., "Minireview: Gut Microbiota: The Neglected Endocrine Organ," *Molecular Endocrinology* 28, no. 8 (August 2014): 1221–38, https://www.ncbi.nlm.nih.gov/pmc/articles/PMC5414803/.

24. Robert Keith Wallace and Samantha Wallace, *Gut Crisis: How Diet, Probiotics, and Friendly Bacteria Help You Lose Weight and Heal Your Body and Mind* (Fairfield, IA: Dharma, 2017), chap. 3, Kindle.

25. Jawara Allen and Cynthia L. Sears, "Impact of the Gut Microbiome on the Genome and Epigenome of Colon Epithelial Cells: Contributions to Colorectal Cancer Development," *Genome Medicine* 11, no. 1 (February 25, 2019): 11, https://www.ncbi.nlm.nih.gov/pmc/articles/PMC6388476/.

CHAPTER 2

1. Chris Kresser, "How to Tell if You Have a Leaky Gut," Chris Kresser, updated April 26, 2019, https://chriskresser.com/how-to-tell-if-you-have-a-leaky-gut/.

2. Perlmutter, *Brain Maker*, 7.

3. Perlmutter, *Brain Maker*, 16–17.

4. "Autoimmune Diseases," National Institute of Allergy and Infectious Diseases, May 2, 2017, https://www.niaid.nih.gov/diseases-conditions/autoimmune-diseases; "The Health Effects of Overweight and Obesity," Centers for Disease Control and Prevention, June 30, 2020, https://www.cdc.gov/healthyweight/effects/index.html.

CHAPTER 3

1. Chutkan, *The Microbiome Solution*, 13.

2. Steven R. Gundry, *The Plant Paradox: The Hidden Dangers in "Healthy" Foods That Cause Disease and Weight Gain* (New York: HarperCollins, 2017), 68–70.

3. Craig M. Hales et al., "Prescription Drug Use Among Adults Aged 40–79 in the United States and Canada," National Center for Health Statistics Brief no. 347, August 2019, https://www.cdc.gov/nchs/products/databriefs/db347.htm.

4. Don Colbert, *Let Food Be Your Medicine: Dietary Changes Proven to Prevent or Reverse Disease* (Franklin, TN: Worthy Books, 2016), xv.

5. Gundry, *The Plant Paradox*, 84.

6. Perlmutter, *Brain Maker*, 53–54.

7. Marcelo Campos, "Leaky Gut: What Is It, and What Does It Mean for You?," Harvard Health, updated October 22, 2019, https://www.health.harvard.edu/blog/leaky-gut-what-is-it-and-what-does-it-mean-for-you-2017092212451.

8. Gundry, *The Plant Paradox*, 68–70.

9. Gundry, *The Plant Paradox*, 20.

10. University of Gothenburg, "Surface Area of the Digestive Tract Much Smaller than Previously Thought," ScienceDaily, April 23, 2014, https://www.sciencedaily.com/releases/2014/04/140423111505.htm.

11. Alessio Fasano and Susie Flaherty, *Gluten Freedom: The Nation's Leading Expert Offers the Essential Guide to a Healthy, Gluten-Free Lifestyle* (Nashville: Wiley General Trade, 2014), 56–57.

12. Matthew Solan, "Putting a Stop to Leaky Gut," Harvard Health, updated November 21, 2018, https://www.health.harvard.edu/blog/putting-a-stop-to-leaky-gut-2018111815289.

CHAPTER 4

1. Don Colbert, *Dr. Colbert's Fasting Zone: Reset Your Health and Cleanse Your Body in 21 Days* (Lake Mary, FL: Siloam, 2020), 44.

2. Ruairi Robertson, "How Your Gut Bacteria Can Influence Your Weight," Healthline, February 13, 2018, https://www.healthline.com/nutrition/gut-bacteria-and-weight#section2.

3. Chutkan, *The Microbiome Solution*, 72.

4. Eili Y. Klein et al., "Global Increase and Geographic Convergence in Antibiotic Consumption Between 2000 and 2015," *Proceedings of*

the National Academy of Sciences 115, no. 15 (April 2018): E3463–70, https://www.pnas.org/content/115/15/E3463.

5. Centers for Disease Control and Prevention, *Antibiotic Use in the United States, 2018 Update: Progress and Opportunities* (Atlanta: US Department of Health and Human Services, CDC, 2019), 3, https://www.cdc.gov/antibiotic-use/stewardship-report/pdf/stewardship-report-2018-508.pdf.

6. Laura M. Cox and Martin J. Blaser, "Antibiotics in Early Life and Obesity," *Nature Reviews: Endocrinology* 11, no. 3 (2015): 182–90, https://www.ncbi.nlm.nih.gov/pmc/articles/PMC4487629/.

7. Chutkan, *The Microbiome Solution*, 39.

8. M. B. Azad et al., "Impact of Maternal Intrapartum Antibiotics, Method of Birth and Breastfeeding on Gut Microbiota During the First Year of Life: A Prospective Cohort Study," *BJOG: An International Journal of Obstetrics and Gynaecology* 123, no. 6 (2016): 983–93, https://obgyn.onlinelibrary.wiley.com/doi/full/10.1111/1471-0528.13601.

9. Pajau Vangay et al., "Antibiotics, Pediatric Dysbiosis, and Disease," *Cell Host and Microbe* 17, no. 5 (2015): 553–64, https://www.ncbi.nlm.nih.gov/pmc/articles/PMC5555213/; Catharina Lavebratt et al., "Early Exposure to Antibiotic Drugs and Risk for Psychiatric Disorders: A Population-Based Study," *Translational Psychiatry* 9, no. 317 (2019), https://www.nature.com/articles/s41398-019-0653-9.

10. Martin J. Blaser, *Missing Microbes: How the Overuse of Antibiotics Is Fueling Our Modern Plagues* (New York: Henry Holt and Company, 2014), 2–6, 178.

11. Enders, *Gut*, 232.

12. Chutkan, *The Microbiome Solution*, 109.

13. Yvette Brazier, "One Course of Antibiotics Disrupts Gut Microbiome for a Year," Medical News Today, November 10, 2015, https://www.medicalnewstoday.com/articles/302179.

14. Gundry, *The Plant Paradox*, 98–101.

15. Centers for Disease Control and Prevention, *Antibiotic Use in the United States, 2018 Update*, 3.

16. Chutkan, *The Microbiome Solution*, 45.

17. Erika Utzeri and Paolo Usai, "Role of Non-steroidal Anti-inflammatory Drugs on Intestinal Permeability and Nonalcoholic Fatty Liver Disease," *World Journal of Gastroenterology* 23, no. 22 (2017): 3954–63, https://www.ncbi.nlm.nih.gov/pmc/articles/PMC5473116/.

18. Gundry, *The Plant Paradox*, 102.

19. Gundry, *The Plant Paradox*, 84.

20. Sung Chul Park et al., "Prevention and Management of Non-steroidal Anti-inflammatory Drugs-Induced Small Intestinal Injury," *World Journal of Gastroenterology* 17, no. 42 (2011): 4647–53, https://www.ncbi.nlm.nih.gov/pmc/articles/PMC3237301/.

21. Chutkan, *The Microbiome Solution*, 52.

22. Carol Grieve, "Leaky Gut: Is It Becoming an Epidemic?," Food Integrity Now, May 27, 2015, https://foodintegritynow.org/leaky-gut-is-it-becoming-an-epidemic/.

23. Carrie Vitt, "Why Stomach Acid Is Good for You and How to Increase It Naturally," Deliciously Organic, September 12, 2016, https://deliciouslyorganic.net/why-stomach-acid-is-good-for-you-increase-naturally/.

24. Gundry, *The Plant Paradox*, 104–5.

25. Mark Volmer, "Low Stomach Acid & Irritable Bowel Syndrome: What's the Connection?," Medium, April 21, 2017, https://medium.com/@Flourish_Clinic/low-stomach-acid-irritable-bowel-syndrome-whats-the-connection-9c67c6d9a5b3.

26. Gundry, *The Plant Paradox*, 105.

27. Gundry, *The Plant Paradox*, 105–6.

28. Mateusz Perkowski, "Adoption of Biotech Alfalfa Lags other GMO Crops," *Capital Press*, updated December 13, 2018, https://www.capitalpress.com/nation_world/nation/adoption-of-biotech-alfalfa-lags-other-gmo-crops/article_8e99ac91-1534-5d03-b0f4-37fd93c6ca14.html.

29. "GMO Crops, Animal Food, and Beyond," US Food and Drug Administration, March 4, 2020, https://www.fda.gov/food/agricultural-biotechnology/gmo-crops-animal-food-and-beyond.

30. "GMO Crops, Animal Food, and Beyond," US Food and Drug Administration.

31. "GMO Crops, Animal Food, and Beyond," US Food and Drug Administration.

32. Stuart Smyth, "How GM Papaya Saved Hawaii's Papaya Industry," SAIFood, June 2, 2015, https://saifood.ca/gm-papaya/.

33. "GMO Crops, Animal Food, and Beyond," US Food and Drug Administration.

34. "GMO Crops, Animal Food, and Beyond," US Food and Drug Administration.

35. Perlmutter, *Brain Maker*, 173; Food Democracy Now! and the Detox Project, *Glyphosate: Unsafe on Any Plate*, 3, accessed August 14, 2020, https://s3.amazonaws.com/media.fooddemocracynow.org/images/FDN_Glyphosate_FoodTesting_Report_p2016.pdf.

36. Edward Group, "GMOs Cause Gut Damage," Global Healing, updated June 8, 2016, https://globalhealing.com/natural-health/gmo-foods-cause-gut-damage-2/.

37. Awad A. Shehata et al., "The Effect of Glyphosate on Potential Pathogens and Beneficial Members of Poultry Microbiota in Vitro," *Current Microbiology* 66, no. 4 (2013): 350–58, https://pubmed.ncbi.nlm.nih.gov/23224412/.

38. Group, "GMOs Cause Gut Damage."

39. Group, "GMOs Cause Gut Damage."

40. Gundry, *The Plant Paradox*, 121–22.

41. Group, "GMOs Cause Gut Damage."

42. Jeffrey M. Smith, "Are Genetically Modified Foods a Gut-Wrenching Combination?," Institute for Responsible Technology, accessed August 14, 2020, https://www.responsibletechnology.org/for-review/glutenintroduction/.

43. Smith, "Are Genetically Modified Foods a Gut-Wrenching Combination?"

44. Carl Schmidt, "GMOs, Leaky Gut, & Inflammation: You Can't Fool Mother Nature," American Autoimmune Related Diseases Association, accessed August 14, 2020, https://www.aarda.org/gmo-foods-leaky-gut-inflammation/.

45. Grieve, "Leaky Gut: Is It Becoming an Epidemic?"

46. Campos, "Leaky Gut: What Is It, and What Does It Mean for You?"; Thomas Jefferson University, "Stronger Intestinal Barrier May Prevent Cancer in the Rest of the Body, New Study Suggests," ScienceDaily, February 21, 2012, https://www.sciencedaily.com/releases/2012/02/120221212345.htm.

47. "GMO Crops, Animal Food, and Beyond," US Food and Drug Administration.

48. Perlmutter, *Brain Maker*, 173.

49. "Chlorine Chemistry: Essential to Safer Water for 100 Years, and Running," American Chemistry Council, accessed August 14, 2020, https://chlorine.americanchemistry.com/Chlorine/Safer-Water/.

50. Lisa Richards, "How Does Chlorine Affect Your Immune System?," The Candida Diet, February 1, 2019, https://www.thecandidadiet.com/chlorine-and-candida/.

51. Pratibha Rialch, "Removing Pesticides from Fruits and Vegetables," Centre for Science and Environment, accessed August 14, 2020, https://www.cseindia.org/removing-pesticides-from-fruits-and-vegetables-2681.

52. Ocean Robbins, "Pesticides in Food: What You Should Know and Why It Matters," Food Revolution Network, September 20, 2019, https://foodrevolution.org/blog/pesticides-facts/.

53. Patricia Cohen, "Roundup Weedkiller Is Blamed for Cancers, but Farmers Say It's Not Going Away," *New York Times*, September 20, 2019, https://www.nytimes.com/2019/09/20/business/bayer-roundup.html.

54. "Pesticide Residues in Food," World Health Organization, February 19, 2018, https://www.who.int/news-room/fact-sheets/detail/pesticide-residues-in-food.

55. Gundry, *The Plant Paradox*, 84.

56. Xianling Yuan et al., "Gut Microbiota: An Underestimated and Unintended Recipient for Pesticide-Induced Toxicity," *Chemosphere* 227 (July 2019): Abstract, https://www.sciencedirect.com/science/article/abs/pii/S0045653519307416.

57. EWG Science Team, "EWG's 2020 Shopper's Guide to Pesticides in Produce," Environmental Working Group, March 25, 2020, https://www.ewg.org/foodnews/summary.php.

58. EWG Science Team, "EWG's 2020 Shopper's Guide to Pesticides in Produce."

59. Maitreyi Raman, Angela Sirounis, and Jennifer Shrubsole, *The Complete Prebiotic & Probiotic Health Guide: A Vegetarian Plan for Balancing Your Gut Flora* (Toronto: Robert Rose, 2015), 44.

60. Centers for Disease Control and Prevention, "Nearly Half a Million Americans Suffered from *Clostridium difficile* Infections in a Single Year," press release, last reviewed March 22, 2017, https://www.cdc.gov/media/releases/2015/p0225-clostridium-difficile.html.

61. Justyna Bien, Vindhya Palagani, and Przemyslaw Bozko, "The Intestinal Microbiota Dysbiosis and *Clostridium difficile* Infection: Is There a Relationship with Inflammatory Bowel Disease?," *Therapeutic Advances*

in Gastroenterology 6, no. 1 (2013): 53–68, https://www.ncbi.nlm.nih.gov/pmc/articles/PMC3539291/.

62. Centers for Disease Control and Prevention, "Nearly Half a Million Americans Suffered from *Clostridium difficile* Infections in a Single Year."

63. Robert Steffen, "Epidemiology of Travellers' Diarrhea," *Journal of Travel Medicine* 24, suppl. 1 (April 1, 2017): S2–S5, https://academic.oup.com/jtm/article/24/suppl_1/S2/3782734.

64. Thad Wilkins and Jacqueline Sequoia, "Probiotics for Gastrointestinal Conditions: A Summary of the Evidence," *American Family Physician* 96, no. 3 (August 1, 2017):170–78, https://www.aafp.org/afp/2017/0801/p170.html.

65. Raman, Sirounis, and Shrubsole, *The Complete Prebiotic & Probiotic Health Guide*, 43.

66. Mary Hickson, "Probiotics in the Prevention of Antibiotic-Associated Diarrhoea and *Clostridium difficile* Infection," *Therapeutic Advances in Gastroenterology* 4, no. 3 (2011): 185–97, https://www.ncbi.nlm.nih.gov/pmc/articles/PMC3105609/.

67. Michelle Moore, "What's the Best *C. Diff* Treatment?," *C. Difficile* Treatment, accessed August 17, 2020, https://www.c-difficile-treatment.com/treatments/.

68. "*C. difficile* Infection," Mayo Clinic, January 4, 2020, https://www.mayoclinic.org/diseases-conditions/c-difficile/diagnosis-treatment/drc-20351697.

69. Moore, "What's the Best *C. Diff* Treatment?"; "*C. difficile* Infection," Mayo Clinic.

CHAPTER 5

1. Furness, Kunze, and Clerc, "Nutrient Tasting and Signaling Mechanisms in the Gut. II. The Intestine as a Sensory Organ."

2. "5 Most Common Food Allergies People Don't Know They Have," The Wellness Way, July 29, 2019, https://thewellnessway.com/most-common-food-allergies/; "Recognizing and Treating Reaction Symptoms," Food Allergy Research and Education, accessed August 17, 2020, https://www.foodallergy.org/resources/recognizing-and-treating-reaction-symptoms.

3. Helen West, "The 8 Most Common Food Allergies," Healthline, January 25, 2017, https://www.healthline.com/nutrition/common-food-allergies.

4. Fasano and Flaherty, *Gluten Freedom*, 54–55.

5. Jill Carnahan, "Zonulin: A Discovery That Changed the Way We View Inflammation, Autoimmune Disease and Cancer," Dr. Jill, July 14, 2013, https://www.jillcarnahan.com/2013/07/14/zonulin-leaky-gut/.

CHAPTER 6

1. Smith, "Are Genetically Modified Foods a Gut-Wrenching Combination?"

2. Perlmutter, *Brain Maker*, 151.

3. Klaas Vandepoele and Yves Van de Peer, "Exploring the Plant Transcriptome through Phylogenetic Profiling," *Plant Physiology* 137, no. 1 (January 2005): 31–42, https://www.ncbi.nlm.nih.gov/pmc/articles/PMC548836/; Perlmutter, *Brain Maker*, 153.

4. Anastasia V. Balakireva and Andrey A Zamyatnin, "Properties of Gluten Intolerance: Gluten Structure, Evolution, Pathogenicity and Detoxification Capabilities," *Nutrients* 8, no. 10 (October 18, 2016): 644, https://www.ncbi.nlm.nih.gov/pmc/articles/PMC5084031/.

5. "Symptoms of Non-Celiac Gluten Sensitivity," Beyond Celiac, accessed August 27, 2020, https://www.beyondceliac.org/celiac-disease/non-celiac-gluten-sensitivity/symptoms/.

6. Justin Hollon et al., "Effect of Gliadin on Permeability of Intestinal Biopsy Explants from Celiac Disease Patients and Patients with Non-celiac Gluten Sensitivity," *Nutrients* 7, no. 3 (February 27, 2015): 1565–76, https://www.ncbi.nlm.nih.gov/pmc/articles/PMC4377866/.

7. Perlmutter, *Brain Maker*, 150–51.

8. Perlmutter, *Brain Maker*, 149.

9. Mark E. M. Obrenovich, "Leaky Gut, Leaky Brain?," *Microorganisms* 6, no. 4 (October 18, 2018): 107, https://www.ncbi.nlm.nih.gov/pmc/articles/PMC6313445/.

10. Gundry, *The Plant Paradox*, 43–44.

11. Carnahan, "Zonulin."

12. Perlmutter, *Brain Maker*, 149.

13. "Lectins: The Gluten-Lectin Leaky Gut Connection," Shield Nutraceuticals, accessed August 18, 2020, https://shieldnutra.com/gluten-lectin-leaky-gut-connection/.

14. Gundry, *The Plant Paradox*, 51.

15. Emeran Mayer, *The Mind-Gut Connection: How the Hidden Conversation Within Our Bodies Impacts Our Mood, Our Choices, and Our Overall Health*, paperback ed. (New York: Harper Wave, 2018), 250.

16. Perlmutter, *Brain Maker*, 55.

17. Gundry, *The Plant Paradox*, 51–52.

18. Mayer, *The Mind-Gut Connection*, 250.

19. Michael Ruscio, *Healthy Gut, Healthy You: The Personalized Plan to Transform Your Health from the Inside Out* (Las Vegas: The Ruscio Institute, 2018), chap. 6, Kindle.

20. Perlmutter, *Brain Maker*, 185.

21. "Facts About IBS," International Foundation for Gastrointestinal Disorders, November 24, 2016, https://aboutibs.org/what-is-ibs/facts-about-ibs-2.html.

22. Perlmutter, *Brain Maker*, 184–85.

23. Chutkan, *The Microbiome Solution*, 128.

24. Chutkan, *The Microbiome Solution*, 125–126.

25. Chutkan, *The Microbiome Solution*, 122.

26. Don Otter and Shelby Anderson, "Five Things Everyone Should Know About…A2 Milk," Wisconsin State Farmer, July 3, 2019, https://www.wisfarmer.com/story/news/2019/07/03/five-things-everyone-should-know-about-a-2-milk/1642645001/.

27. Linni Kral, "The Health Battle Behind America's Next Milk Trend," *The Atlantic*, January 27, 2017, https://www.theatlantic.com/science/archive/2017/01/a-tale-of-two-milks/514397/.

28. Maureen E. Taylor et al., "Discovery and Classification of Glycan-Binding Proteins," in *Essentials of Glycobiology* [Internet], 3rd ed., ed. Ajit Varki et al. (Cold Spring Harbor, NY: Cold Spring Harbor Laboratory Press; 2017), https://www.ncbi.nlm.nih.gov/books/NBK453061/.

29. "Lectins," Shield Nutraceuticals.

30. Gundry, *The Plant Paradox*, 8–11.

31. Steven Gundry, "Your Definitive Guide to Lectins," Dr. Gundry, accessed August 18, 2020, https://drgundry.com/lectin-guide/; "How Do You Know If You Are Sensitive to Lectins?," Vibrant Wellness, accessed August 18, 2020, https://www.vibrant-wellness.com/how-do-you-know-if-you-are-sensitive-to-lectins/.

32. Gundry, *The Plant Paradox*, 15–17, 206.

33. Gundry MD Team, "15 Steps to Reduce Lectins in Your Diet," Gundry MD, May 23, 2017, https://gundrymd.com/reduce-lectins-diet/.

34. David L. J. Freed, "Do Dietary Lectins Cause Disease?," *BMJ* 318, no. 7190 (April 17, 1999): 1023–24, https://www.ncbi.nlm.nih.gov/pmc/articles/PMC1115436/.

35. Gundry, *The Plant Paradox*, 76.

36. "Lectins," Shield Nutraceuticals.

37. Gundry, *The Plant Paradox*, 21.

38. "Lectins," Shield Nutraceuticals.

39. Gundry, *The Plant Paradox*, 237.

40. Jordan Reasoner, "How to Properly Prepare Beans (So They're Gut-Healthy)," Healthy Gut, updated January 8, 2019, https://healthygut.com/articles/how-to-properly-prepare-beans/.

41. Ryan Andrews, "All About Lectins," Precision Nutrition, accessed August 19, 2020, https://www.precisionnutrition.com/all-about-lectins.

42. Wendy Myers, "Complete List of Artificial Sweeteners," Myers Detox, accessed August 19, 2020, https://myersdetox.com/complete-list-of-artificial-sweeteners/.

43. Xiaoming Bian et al., "The Artificial Sweetener Acesulfame Potassium Affects the Gut Microbiome and Body Weight Gain in CD-1 Mice," *PloS One* 12, no. 6 (June 8, 2017): e0178426, https://www.ncbi.nlm.nih.gov/pmc/articles/PMC5464538/.

44. Myers, "Complete List of Artificial Sweeteners."

45. Joseph Mercola, "Science Review Reveals Laundry List of Health Hazards Associated with Splenda Consumption," Mercola, December 18, 2013, https://articles.mercola.com/sites/articles/archive/2013/12/18/sucralose-side-effects.aspx.

46. "Gas/Bloating," GI Health, accessed August 19, 2020, https://mygi.health/education/symptoms/bloating.

47. Jotham Suez et al., "Artificial Sweeteners Induce Glucose Intolerance by Altering the Gut Microbiota," *Nature* 514, no. 7521 (2014): 181–86, https://pubmed.ncbi.nlm.nih.gov/25231862/.

48. "19 Notable High Fructose Corn Syrup Statistics," Health Research Funding, accessed August 19, 2020, https://healthresearchfunding.org/19-notable-high-fructose-corn-syrup-statistics/.

49. Miriam B. Vos and Joel E. Lavine, "Dietary Fructose in Nonalcoholic Fatty Liver Disease," *Hepatology* 57, no. 6 (June 2013): 2525–31, https://

aasldpubs.onlinelibrary.wiley.com/doi/full/10.1002/hep.26299; Lea M. D. Delbridge et al., "Diabetic Cardiomyopathy: The Case for a Role of Fructose in Disease Etiology," *Diabetes* 65, no. 12 (December 2016): 3521–28, https://diabetes.diabetesjournals.org/content/65/12/3521.

50. Hunter Myüz and Michael C. Hout, "Trick or Treat? How Artificial Sweeteners Affect the Brain and Body," *Frontiers for Young Minds*, March 29, 2019, https://kids.frontiersin.org/article/10.3389/frym.2019.00051.

51. "19 Notable High Fructose Corn Syrup Statistics," Health Research Funding.

52. Mayer, *The Mind-Gut Connection*, 248.

53. D. Partridge et al., "Food Additives: Assessing the Impact of Exposure to Permitted Emulsifiers on Bowel and Metabolic Health—Introducing the FADiets Study," *Nutrition Bulletin* 44, no. 4 (2019): 329–49, https://www.ncbi.nlm.nih.gov/pmc/articles/PMC6899614/; Sarah Kay Hoffman, "Your Guide to Emulsifiers in Food," A Gutsy Girl, accessed August 19, 2020, https://agutsygirl.com/2020/06/12/your-guide-to-emulsifiers-in-food/.

54. HealthDay News, "Cheap Processed Foods Making Americans Obese, Unhealthy," United Press International, January 10, 2020, https://www.upi.com/Health_News/2020/01/10/Cheap-processed-foods-making-Americans-obese-unhealthy/5161578627200/.

55. Andrew Orr, "Food Additives and Emulsifiers May Increase Inflammation and Anxiety," Dr. Andrew Orr, January 29, 2019, https://drandreworr.com.au/food-additives-and-emulsifiers-may-increase-inflammation-and-anxiety/.

56. "Saturated Fat," American Heart Association, accessed August 19, 2020, https://www.heart.org/en/healthy-living/healthy-eating/eat-smart/fats/saturated-fats.

57. Perlmutter, *Brain Maker*, 56.

58. Julie A. Gegner, Richard J. Ulevitch, and Peter S. Tobias, "Lipopolysaccharide (LPS) Signal Transduction and Clearance: Dual Roles for LPS Binding Protein and Membrane CD14," *Journal of Biological Chemistry* 270, no. 10 (1995): 5320–25, https://www.jbc.org/content/270/10/5320.long.

59. Perlmutter, *Brain Maker*, 57.

60. Matt Lehrer, "What Are Lipopolysaccharides (LPS)?," SelfHacked, January 17, 2020, https://selfhacked.com/blog/lipopolysaccharides/.

61. Perlmutter, *Brain Maker*, 57, 59.

62. Gundry, *The Plant Paradox*, 64–65.

63. Richard Hagmeyer, "What Are Lipopolysaccharides, and How Can They Affect Thyroid Health?," Dr. Hagmeyer, August 25, 2014, https://drhagmeyer.com/what-are-lipopolysaccharides-and-how-can-they-affect-thyroid-health/.

64. Marius Trøseid et al., "Plasma Lipopolysaccharide Is Closely Associated with Glycemic Control and Abdominal Obesity: Evidence from Bariatric Surgery," *Diabetes Care* 36, no. 11 (2013): 3627–32, https://www.ncbi.nlm.nih.gov/pmc/articles/PMC3816876/.

65. Kelton Tremellen, Natalie McPhee, and Karma Pearce, "Metabolic Endotoxaemia Related Inflammation Is Associated with Hypogonadism in Overweight Men," *Basic and Clinical Andrology* 27, no. 5 (2017), https://www.ncbi.nlm.nih.gov/pmc/articles/PMC5341351/.

66. Brian K. McFarlin et al., "Oral Spore-Based Probiotic Supplementation Was Associated with Reduced Incidence of Post-prandial Dietary Endotoxin, Triglycerides, and Disease Risk Biomarkers," *World Journal of Gastrointestinal Pathophysiology* 8, no. 3 (2017): 117–26, https://www.ncbi.nlm.nih.gov/pmc/articles/PMC5561432/.

67. Perlmutter, *Brain Maker*, 151.

68. "Constipation," Mayo Clinic, June 29, 2019, https://www.mayoclinic.org/diseases-conditions/constipation/symptoms-causes/syc-20354253.

69. "Constipation," Mayo Clinic.

70. Adil Bharucha, John H. Pemberton, and G. Richard Locke III, "American Gastroenterological Association Technical Review on Constipation," *Gastroenterology* 144, no. 1 (January 2013): 218–38, https://www.ncbi.nlm.nih.gov/pmc/articles/PMC3531555/.

71. "Constipation," Johns Hopkins Medicine, accessed August 19, 2020, https://www.hopkinsmedicine.org/health/conditions-and-diseases/constipation; Thomas Sommers et al., "Emergency Department Burden of Constipation in the United States from 2006 to 2011," *American Journal of Gastroenterology* 110, no. 4 (April 2015): 572–79, https://pubmed.ncbi.nlm.nih.gov/25803399/.

72. Ruscio, *Healthy Gut, Healthy You*, chap. 13, Kindle.

73. Enders, *Gut*, 109.

74. Yvonne Oligschlaeger et al., "Inflammatory Bowel Disease: A Stressed 'Gut/Feeling,'" *Cells* 8, no. 7 (June 30, 2019): 659, https://www.ncbi.nlm.nih.gov/pmc/articles/PMC6678997/.

75. Perlmutter, *Brain Maker*, 85.

76. "*Bifidobacterium infantis*: Major Benefits, Food Sources and Its Role in Weight Loss," Billion Cheers, June 14, 2019, https://billioncheers.com/blog/bifidobacterium-infantis/.

77. Enders, *Gut*, 226.

78. Rahimah Herd, "What Is the Skin Microbiome? (Plus, What It Means for Clearer, Healthier Skin)," Dermstore, April 6, 2020, https://www.dermstore.com/blog/top_ten/what-is-skin-microbiome/.

79. Enders, *Gut*, 226.

CHAPTER 7

1. "The Health Effects of Overweight and Obesity," Centers for Disease Control and Prevention.

CHAPTER 8

1. "Acid Reflux: Overview," American College of Gastroenterology, accessed August 20, 2020, https://gi.org/topics/acid-reflux/.

2. Dorathy Gass, "10 Signs and Symptoms of G.E.R.D. (Acid Reflux)," RMHealthy, January 19, 2018, https://rmhealthy.com/10-signs-symptoms-g-e-r-d-acid-reflux/.

3. Nancy Kushner and Robert Kushner, "Obesity and Heartburn: What Is the Link?," Obesity Action Coalition, Winter 2013, https://www.obesityaction.org/community/article-library/obesity-heartburn-what-is-the-link/.

4. Jai Moo Shin and George Sachs, "Pharmacology of Proton Pump Inhibitors," *Current Gastroenterology Reports* 10, no. 6 (2008): 528–34, https://www.ncbi.nlm.nih.gov/pmc/articles/PMC2855237/.

5. Kristina Sauerwein, "Heartburn Drugs Linked to Fatal Heart and Kidney Disease, Stomach Cancer," Washington University School of Medicine, May 30, 2019, https://medicine.wustl.edu/news/popular-heartburn-drugs-linked-to-fatal-heart-disease-chronic-kidney-disease-stomach-cancer/; Avinash K. Nehra et al., "Proton Pump Inhibitors: Review of Emerging Concerns," *Mayo Clinic Proceedings, Concise Review for Clinicians* 93, no. 2 (February 1, 2018): 240–46, https://www.mayoclinicproceedings.org/article/S0025-6196(17)30841-8/fulltext.

6. Koichiro Matsuo and Jeffrey B. Palmer, "Anatomy and Physiology of Feeding and Swallowing: Normal and Abnormal," *Physical Medicine*

and Rehabilitation Clinics of North America 19, no. 4 (2008): 691–707, vii, https://www.ncbi.nlm.nih.gov/pmc/articles/PMC2597750/.

7. Matsuo and Palmer, "Anatomy and Physiology of Feeding and Swallowing"; Jose Vega, "How Your Brain Controls Swallowing," Verywell Health, January 2, 2020, https://www.verywellhealth.com/how-do-our-brains-control-swallowing-3146398.

8. Enders, *Gut*, 95–96.

9. Jonathan V. Wright and Lane Lenard, *Why Stomach Acid Is Good for You: Natural Relief from Heartburn, Indigestion, Reflux, & GERD* (Lanham, MD: M. Evans, 2001), 41.

10. "Acid Reflux: FAQs," American College of Gastroenterology, accessed August 20, 2020, https://gi.org/topics/acid-reflux/#tabs3.

11. Mark Henricks, "What Is GERD? Symptoms, Causes, Diagnosis, Treatment, and Prevention," Everyday Health, August 12, 2020, https://www.everydayhealth.com/gerd/guide/.

12. "Heartburn and Foods: Dos and Don'ts," Everyday Health, accessed August 20, 2020, https://www.everydayhealth.com/digestive-health-pictures/heartburn-and-foods-dos-and-donts.aspx.

13. Sharon Gillson, "10 Things to Stop Doing If You Have GERD," Verywell Health, July 23, 2020, https://www.verywellhealth.com/stop-doing-with-gerd-1742213.

14. "Heartburn and Foods," Everyday Health.

15. "Heartburn and Foods," Everyday Health.

16. Henricks, "What Is GERD? Symptoms, Causes, Diagnosis, Treatment, and Prevention."

17. Gillson, "10 Things to Stop Doing If You Have GERD."

18. "Heartburn: The Food Allergy Connection?," Paleo Leap, accessed August 20, 2020, https://paleoleap.com/heartburn-food-allergy-connection/.

19. Henricks, "What Is GERD? Symptoms, Causes, Diagnosis, Treatment, and Prevention."

20. "A Complete Guide to Viagra® (Sildenafil) Side Effects," Hims, updated May 12, 2020, https://www.forhims.com/blog/a-complete-guide-viagra-sildenafil-side-effects; "A Complete Guide to Cialis (Tadalafil) Side Effects," Hims, updated June 21, 2020, https://www.forhims.com/blog/a-complete-guide-cialis-tadalafil-side-effects; Sharon Gillson, "Causes and Risk Factors of Gastroesophageal Reflux Disease (GERD)," Verywell

Health, August 12, 2019, https://www.verywellhealth.com/what-causes-gerd-1741914.

21. Gillson, "Causes and Risk Factors of Gastroesophageal Reflux Disease (GERD)."

22. Gillson, "10 Things to Stop Doing If You Have GERD."

23. Gillson, "10 Things to Stop Doing If You Have GERD."

24. Benjamin Thong, Soelaiman Ima-Nirwana, and Kok-Yong Chin, "Proton Pump Inhibitors and Fracture Risk: A Review of Current Evidence and Mechanisms Involved," *International Journal of Environmental Research and Public Health* 16, no. 9 (May 2019): 1571, https://www.ncbi.nlm.nih.gov/pmc/articles/PMC6540255/.

25. Sascha Kopic and John P. Geibel, "Gastric Acid, Calcium Absorption, and Their Impact on Bone Health," *Physiological Reviews* 93, no. 1 (2013): 189–268, https://journals.physiology.org/doi/full/10.1152/physrev.00015.2012.

26. Chutkan, *The Microbiome Solution*, 51.

27. Wright and Lenard, *Why Stomach Acid Is Good for You*, 22.

28. Stephen D. Krasinski et al., "Fundic Atrophic Gastritis in an Elderly Population. Effect on Hemoglobin and Several Serum Nutritional Indicators," *Journal of the American Geriatrics Society* 34, no. 11 (November 1986): 800–6, https://pubmed.ncbi.nlm.nih.gov/3771980/.

29. Giovanni Bruno et al., "Proton Pump Inhibitors and Dysbiosis: Current Knowledge and Aspects to Be Clarified," *World Journal of Gastroenterology* 25, no. 22 (2019): 2706–19, https://www.ncbi.nlm.nih.gov/pmc/articles/PMC6580352/.

30. "Digestive Diseases," National Center for Health Statistics, Centers for Disease Control and Prevention, March 1, 2019, https://www.cdc.gov/nchs/fastats/digestive-diseases.htm.

31. "Peptic Ulcers," Kids Health, July 2015, https://teenshealth.org/en/parents/peptic-ulcers.html.

32. "Peptic Ulcer," Mayo Clinic, August 6, 2020, https://www.mayoclinic.org/diseases-conditions/peptic-ulcer/symptoms-causes/syc-20354223.

33. "What Causes Stomach Cancer?," American Cancer Society, revised December 14, 2017, https://www.cancer.org/cancer/stomach-cancer/causes-risks-prevention/what-causes.html.

34. Enders, *Gut*, 206–7.

35. Wright and Lenard, *Why Stomach Acid Is Good for You*, 92.

36. "Peptic Ulcers," Kids Health.

37. "Peptic Ulcers," Kids Health; "Peptic Ulcer," Mayo Clinic.

38. "Peptic Ulcer," Mayo Clinic.

39. Wright and Lenard, *Why Stomach Acid Is Good for You*, 153–54.

40. Wright and Lenard, *Why Stomach Acid Is Good for You*, 92–94.

41. Ryuzo Deguchi et al., "Effect of Pretreatment with *Lactobacillus gasseri* OLL2716 on First-Line *Helicobacter pylori* Eradication Therapy," *Journal of Gastroenterology and Hepatology* 27, no. 5 (2012): 888–92, https://www.ncbi.nlm.nih.gov/pmc/articles/PMC3504346/.

42. Ami D. Sperber, "IBS and Non-GI Functional Disorders," International Foundation for Gastrointestinal Disorders, updated September 8, 2016, https://www.aboutibs.org/other-disorders/ibs-and-non-gi-functional-disorders.html.

43. Robin Spiller, "Post Infectious IBS," International Foundation for Gastrointestinal Disorders, updated June 15, 2016, https://www.aboutibs.org/what-is-ibs-sidenav/post-infectious-ibs.html.

44. "Irritable Bowel Syndrome," American College of Gastroenterology, accessed August 20, 2020, https://gi.org/topics/irritable-bowel-syndrome/.

45. Brian E. Lacy, *Making Sense of IBS: A Physician Answers Your Questions about Irritable Bowel Syndrome*, 2nd ed. (Baltimore: Johns Hopkins University Press, 2013), 25.

46. Lacy, *Making Sense of IBS*, 138–143.

47. Peter Whorwell, *Take Control of Your IBS: The Complete Guide to Managing Your Symptoms* (London: Vermilion, 2017), table 9.

48. Jane Anderson, "Differentiating Between IBS, Celiac Disease, and Gluten Sensitivity," Verywell Health, October 2, 2019, https://www.verywellhealth.com/gluten-vs-irritable-bowel-syndrome-562696. .

49. "Small Intestinal Bacterial Overgrowth (SIBO)," Mayo Clinic, February 28, 2020, https://www.mayoclinic.org/diseases-conditions/small-intestinal-bacterial-overgrowth/symptoms-causes/syc-20370168.

50. Askin Erdogan and Satish S. C. Rao, "Small Intestinal Fungal Overgrowth," *Current Gastroenterology Reports* 17, no. 4 (2015): 16, https://pubmed.ncbi.nlm.nih.gov/25786900/.

51. Oreoluwa Ogunyemi, "Everything About SIBO: Causes, Symptoms, and More," SIBO Survivor, March 12, 2020, https://sibosurvivor.com/what-is-sibo/.

52. "Facts About IBS," International Foundation for Gastrointestinal Disorders, updated November 24, 2016, https://www.aboutibs.org/facts-about-ibs.html.

53. Erdogan and Rao, "Small Intestinal Fungal Overgrowth."

54. "Irritable Bowel Syndrome (IBS) Patients Struggle with Diagnosis, Unhappy with Healthcare Providers," Health Union, April 12, 2017, https://health-union.com/news/ibs-in-america-survey-finds-patients-struggle-with-diagnosis/.

55. Jane Recker, "Scientists Find a Possible Link Between Gut Bacteria and Depression," *Smithsonian Magazine*, February 5, 2019, https://www.smithsonianmag.com/science-nature/scientists-find-possible-link-between-gut-bacteria-and-depression-180971411/.

56. Wright and Lenard, *Why Stomach Acid Is Good for You*, 39–40.

57. Jill Seladi-Schulman, "What Is SIFO, and How Can It Affect Your Gut Health?," Healthline, December 4, 2019, https://www.healthline.com/health/sifo#what-is-sifo.

58. Barbara Bolen, "Small Intestinal Fungal Overgrowth," Verywell Health, September 25, 2019, https://www.verywellhealth.com/small-intestinal-fungal-overgrowth-1945218.

59. "Irritable Bowel Syndrome," Mayo Clinic, March 17, 2018, https://www.mayoclinic.org/diseases-conditions/irritable-bowel-syndrome/symptoms-causes/syc-20360016; "Is This IBS?," IBS Network, accessed August 21, 2020, https://www.theibsnetwork.org/have-i-got-ibs/is-this-ibs/; Lana Burgess, "10 Signs and Symptoms of Irritable Bowel Syndrome," Medical News Today, January 23, 2019, https://www.medicalnewstoday.com/articles/324259.

60. Mi Young Yoon and Sang Sun Yoon, "Disruption of the Gut Ecosystem by Antibiotics," *Yonsei Medical Journal* 59, no. 1 (2018): 4–12, https://www.ncbi.nlm.nih.gov/pmc/articles/PMC5725362/; Amy Myers, "How Antibiotics Affect Your Gut Health," Amy Myers, MD, updated August 11, 2020, https://www.amymyersmd.com/article/antibiotics-gut/.

61. Michael Ruscio, "Everything You Need to Know About SIFO (Small Intestinal Fungal Overgrowth)," *Dr. Ruscio Blog*, December 7, 2019, https://drruscio.com/everything-need-know-sifo-small-intestinal-fungal-overgrowth/; "Small Intestinal Bacterial Overgrowth (SIBO)," Mayo Clinic.

62. "Small Intestinal Bacterial Overgrowth (SIBO)," Mayo Clinic.

63. Lacy, *Making Sense of IBS*, 150.

64. Rajsree Nambudripad, "Do You Have SIBO?," OC Integrative Medicine, accessed August 21, 2020, https://oc-integrative-medicine.com/do-you-have-sibo/.

65. "Small Intestinal Bacterial Overgrowth (SIBO)," Mayo Clinic.

66. Lacy, *Making Sense of IBS*, 150.

67. "What Causes SIBO?—Genetics," SIBO Testing Clinic, November 16, 2015, https://sibotesting.com/what-causes-sibo-genetics/.

68. Lacy, *Making Sense of IBS*, 150.

69. "Small Intestinal Bacterial Overgrowth (SIBO)," Mayo Clinic.

70. Amy Myers, "10 Signs You Have SIBO—Small Intestinal Bacterial Overgrowth," Amy Myers, MD, updated August 11, 2020, https://www.amymyersmd.com/article/sibo-small-intestinal-bacterial-overgrowth-symptoms/.

71. Lacy, *Making Sense of IBS*, 150.

72. Lacy, *Making Sense of IBS*, 150; Ruscio, "Everything You Need to Know About SIFO (Small Intestinal Fungal Overgrowth)."

73. Bharucha, Pemberton, and Locke, "American Gastroenterological Association Technical Review on Constipation."

74. Ruscio, *Healthy Gut, Healthy You*, chap. 2, Kindle.

75. Matthew Murphy, "The Definitive Guide to Small Intestinal Fungal Overgrowth (SIFO)," Happy Mammoth, December 11, 2018, https://happymammoth.co/definitive-guide-to-sifo/.

76. René E. Cormier, "Chapter 90: Abdominal Gas," in *Clinical Methods: The History, Physical, and Laboratory Examinations*, 3rd ed., ed. H. Kenneth Walker, W. Dallas Hall, and J. Willis Hurst (Boston: Butterworths, 1990), https://www.ncbi.nlm.nih.gov/books/NBK417/.

77. Sahar Karimi et al., "The Antimicrobial Activity of Probiotic Bacteria *Escherichia coli* Isolated from Different Natural Sources against Hemorrhagic *E. coli* O157:H7," *Electronic Physician* 10, no. 3 (March 25, 2018): 6548–53, https://www.ncbi.nlm.nih.gov/pmc/articles/PMC5942577/; Anne Trafton, "Probiotics and Antibiotics Create a Killer Combination," MIT News, October 17, 2018, http://news.mit.edu/2018/probiotics-antibiotics-kill-drug-resistant-bacteria-1017.

78. Ruscio, *Healthy Gut, Healthy You*, 173–74.

79. "Celiac Disease: Fast Facts," Beyond Celiac, accessed August 21, 2020, https://www.beyondceliac.org/celiac-disease/facts-and-figures/.

80. Jane Anderson, "How Many People Have Gluten Sensitivity?," Verywell Health, updated June 18, 2019, https://www.verywellhealth.com/how-many-people-have-gluten-sensitivity-562965.

81. "Center for Celiac Research: Celiac Disease FAQ," Massachusetts General for Children, October 7, 2019, https://www.massgeneral.org/children/celiac-disease/faq.

82. "Celiac Disease," WebMD, July 7, 2020, https://www.webmd.com/digestive-disorders/celiac-disease/celiac-disease#1; Becky Bell, "Does Gluten Cause Leaky Gut Syndrome?," Healthline, December 8, 2016, https://www.healthline.com/nutrition/gluten-leaky-gut.

83. "Celiac Disease," WebMD.

84. Chutkan, *The Microbiome Solution*, 76.

85. Jonas F. Ludvigsson et al., "Celiac Disease and Risk of Subsequent Type 1 Diabetes: A General Population Cohort Study of Children and Adolescents," *Diabetes Care* 29, no. 11 (2006): 2483–88, https://care.diabetesjournals.org/content/29/11/2483.

86. Ernie Hood, "Measuring Autoimmunity in America," *Environmental Factor*, April 2018, https://factor.niehs.nih.gov/2018/4/science-highlights/autoimmunity/index.htm.

87. Melissa Conrad Stöppler, "Colitis: Symptoms and Signs," MedicineNet, September 10, 2019, https://www.medicinenet.com/colitis_symptoms_and_signs/symptoms.htm.

88. "Ulcerative Colitis," Mayo Clinic, December 24, 2019, https://www.mayoclinic.org/diseases-conditions/ulcerative-colitis/symptoms-causes/syc-20353326.

89. "Difference Between Colitis and Ulcerative Colitis," Pediaa, September 1, 2016, https://pediaa.com/difference-between-colitis-and-ulcerative-colitis/.

90. "Ulcerative Colitis," Mayo Clinic.

91. Lacy, *Making Sense of IBS*, 160–63.

92. Timothy Huzar, "What Is the Difference Between IBS and IBD?," Medical News Today, November 22, 2018, https://www.medicalnewstoday.com/articles/323778.

93. Michael Kerr and Kristeen Cherney, "The Difference Between Crohn's, UC, and IBD," Healthline, May 11, 2020, https://www.healthline.com/health/crohns-disease/crohns-ibd-uc-difference#ibd.

94. Antonio Di Sario et al.," Biologic Drugs in Crohn's Disease and Ulcerative Colitis: Safety Profile," *Current Drug Safety* 11, no. 1 (2016): 55–61, https://pubmed.ncbi.nlm.nih.gov/26882354/.

95. "Fact Sheet: Biologics," Crohn's and Colitis Foundation, October 2018, https://www.crohnscolitisfoundation.org/sites/default/files/legacy/assets/pdfs/biologic-therapy.pdf.

96. Kerr and Cherney, "The Difference Between Crohn's, UC, and IBD."

97. "Inflammatory Bowel Disease," Mayo Clinic, March 3, 2020, https://www.mayoclinic.org/diseases-conditions/inflammatory-bowel-disease/symptoms-causes/syc-20353315.

98. Kerr and Cherney, "The Difference Between Crohn's, UC, and IBD."

99. Michael O. Schroeder, "Death by Prescription," *U.S. News and World Report*, September 27, 2016, https://health.usnews.com/health-news/patient-advice/articles/2016-09-27/the-danger-in-taking-prescribed-medications.

100. Chutkan, *The Microbiome Solution*, 68.

101. "Crohn's Disease," Mayo Clinic, December 24, 2019, https://www.mayoclinic.org/diseases-conditions/crohns-disease/symptoms-causes/syc-20353304.

102. "Inflammatory Bowel Disease: Data and Statistics," Centers for Disease Control and Prevention, March 21, 2019, https://www.cdc.gov/ibd/data-statistics.htm.

103. Andrews, "All About Lectins."

104. "Crohn's Disease," Mayo Clinic.

105. "Inflammatory Bowel Disease," Mayo Clinic.

106. "Causes of Crohn's Disease," Crohn's and Colitis Foundation, accessed August 22, 2020, https://www.crohnscolitisfoundation.org/what-is-crohns-disease/causes.

107. "Crohn's Disease," Mayo Clinic.

108. Amber J. Tresca, "Crohn's Disease: Causes and Risk Factors," January 23, 2020, https://www.verywellhealth.com/crohns-disease-causes-and-risk-factors-4164358.

109. Sarah Knapton, "Crohn's Disease in Teens Jumps 300 Percent in 10 Years Fuelled by Junk Food," *The Telegraph*, June 18, 2014, https://www.telegraph.co.uk/news/science/science-news/10908884/Crohns-disease-in-teens-jumps-300-per-cent-in-10-years-fuelled-by-junk-food.html.

110. J. Todd Kuenstner et al., "The Consensus from the *Mycobacterium avium ssp paratuberculosis* (MAP) Conference 2017," *Frontiers in Public Health* 275 (September 27, 2017), https://www.frontiersin.org/articles/10.3389/fpubh.2017.00208/full.

111. Kerr and Cherney, "The Difference Between Crohn's, UC, and IBD."

112. "Prof. Thomas Borody," Centre for Digestive Diseases, accessed August 22, 2020, https://centrefordigestivediseases.com/team/prof-thomas-borody/.

113. Carpenter, "That Gut Feeling."

114. Sigrid Breit et al., "Vagus Nerve as Modulator of the Brain-Gut Axis in Psychiatric and Inflammatory Disorders," *Frontiers in Psychiatry* 9, no. 44 (March 13, 2018), https://www.ncbi.nlm.nih.gov/pmc/articles/PMC5859128/; Jordan Rosenfeld, "9 Fascinating Facts About the Vagus Nerve," Mental Floss, November 13, 2018, https://www.mentalfloss.com/article/65710/9-nervy-facts-about-vagus-nerve.

115. "Anxiety Disorders," Office on Women's Health, U.S. Department of Health and Human Services, updated January 30, 2019, https://www.womenshealth.gov/mental-health/mental-health-conditions/anxiety-disorders/.

116. Amy Morin, "Depression Statistics Everyone Should Know," Verywell Mind, March 21, 2020, https://www.verywellmind.com/depression-statistics-everyone-should-know-4159056.

117. Carpenter, "That Gut Feeling."

118. Raphael Kellman, *The Microbiome Breakthrough: Harness the Power of Your Gut Bacteria to Boost Your Mood and Heal Your Body* (New York: Da Capo Press, 2018), 113–14.

119. Perlmutter, *Brain Maker*, 75–79.

120. Kellman, *The Microbiome Breakthrough*, 109.

121. Kellman, *The Microbiome Breakthrough*, 109–14.

122. Amy C. Brown and Ana Valiere, "Probiotics and Medical Nutrition Therapy," *Nutrition in Clinical Care: An Official Publication of Tufts University* 7, no. 2 (2004): 56–68, https://www.ncbi.nlm.nih.gov/pmc/articles/PMC1482314/.

123. Michael Ruscio, "Leaky Gut Supplements," *Dr. Ruscio Blog*, April 6, 2020, https://drruscio.com/leaky-gut-supplements/.

124. Lucía Diez-Guitérrez et al., "Gamma-aminobutyric Acid and Probiotics: Multiple Health Benefits and Their Future in the Global Functional Food and Nutraceuticals Market," *Journal of Functional*

Foods 64 (January 2020), https://www.sciencedirect.com/science/article/pii/S1756464619305936.

125. Emily Deans, "Probiotics for Depression," *Psychology Today*, February 21, 2016, https://www.psychologytoday.com/us/blog/evolutionary-psychiatry/201602/probiotics-depression.

126. Julio Plaza-Díaz et al., "Evidence of the Anti-Inflammatory Effects of Probiotics and Synbiotics in Intestinal Chronic Diseases," *Nutrients* 9, no. 6 (May 28, 2017): 555, https://www.ncbi.nlm.nih.gov/pmc/articles/PMC5490534/.

127. Deans, "Probiotics for Depression."

128. Kellman, *The Microbiome Breakthrough*, 113–14.

129. Díaz et al., "Evidence of the Anti-Inflammatory Effects of Probiotics and Synbiotics in Intestinal Chronic Diseases."

130. Huiyning Wang et al., "Effect of Probiotics on Central Nervous System Functions in Animals and Humans: A Systematic Review," *Journal of Neurogastroenterology and Motility* 22, no. 4 (2016): 589–605, https://www.ncbi.nlm.nih.gov/pmc/articles/PMC5056568/.

131. "ADHD Throughout the Years," Centers for Disease Control and Prevention, March 31, 2020, https://www.cdc.gov/ncbddd/adhd/timeline.html.

132. "General Prevalence of ADHD," Children and Adults with Attention-Deficit/Hyperactivity Disorder (CHADD), accessed August 22, 2020, https://chadd.org/about-adhd/general-prevalence/.

133. Sam Blanchard, "Babies Born by C-Section Are 33% More Likely to Develop Autism and Face a Higher Risk of Having ADHD, Study Claims," *Daily Mail*, updated August 29, 2019, https://www.dailymail.co.uk/health/article-7402667/Babies-born-C-section-33-cent-likely-develop-autism.html.

134. Perlmutter, *Brain Maker*, 93.

135. Diez-Guitérrez et al., "Gamma-aminobutyric Acid and Probiotics."

136. Richard A. Edden et al., "Reduced GABA Concentration in Attention-Deficit/Hyperactivity Disorder," *Archives of General Psychiatry* 69, no. 7 (2012): 750–53, https://www.ncbi.nlm.nih.gov/pmc/articles/PMC3970207/; Perlmutter, *Brain Maker*, 93–94.

137. Perlmutter, *Brain Maker*, 94.

138. "What Is Autism Spectrum Disorder?," Centers for Disease Control and Prevention, March 25, 2020, https://www.cdc.gov/ncbddd/autism/facts.html.

139. Matthew J. Maenner et al., "Prevalence of Autism Spectrum Disorder Among Children Aged 8 Years—Autism and Developmental Disabilities Monitoring Network, 11 Sites, United States, 2016," *Surveillance Summaries* 69, no. 4 (March 27, 2020): 1–12, https://www.cdc.gov/mmwr/volumes/69/ss/ss6904a1.htm?s_cid=ss6904a1_w.

140. "Facts and Statistics," Autism Society, accessed August 23, 2020, https://www.autism-society.org/what-is/facts-and-statistics/.

141. Maenner et al., "Prevalence of Autism Spectrum Disorder Among Children Aged 8 Years."

142. Marina Sarris, "What Causes GI Problems in Autism?," Interactive Autism Network, December 3, 2015, https://iancommunity.org/ssc/what-causes-gi-problems-autism.

143. Timothy Buie et al., "Evaluation, Diagnosis, and Treatment of Gastrointestinal Disorders in Individuals with ASDs: A Consensus Report," *Pediatrics* 125, suppl. 1 (January 2010): S1–S18, https://pediatrics.aappublications.org/content/125/Supplement_1/S1.long.

144. Perlmutter, *Brain Maker*, 119–30.

145. Kellman, *The Microbiome Breakthrough*, 110.

146. Perlmutter, *Brain Maker*, 128.

147. Kristeen Cherney and Ana Gotter, "The 5 Stages of Parkinson's," Healthline, March 29, 2020, https://www.healthline.com/health/parkinsons/stages.

148. "Alzheimer's and Dementia: Facts and Figures," Alzheimer's Association, accessed August 23, 2020, https://www.alz.org/alzheimers-dementia/facts-figures.

149. "What Is Dementia?," Centers for Disease Control and Prevention, April 5, 2019, https://www.cdc.gov/aging/dementia/index.html.

150. "Statistics," Parkinson's Foundation, accessed August 23, 2020, https://www.parkinson.org/Understanding-Parkinsons/Statistics.

151. Perlmutter, *Brain Maker*, 55.

152. Mark E. M. Obrenovich, "Leaky Gut, Leaky Brain?," *Microorganisms* 6, no. 4 (October 18, 2018): 107, https://www.ncbi.nlm.nih.gov/pmc/articles/PMC6313445/.

153. Elizaveta Boitsova et al., "The Inhibitory Effect of LPS on the Expression of GPR81 Lactate Receptor in Blood-Brain Barrier Model in Vitro," *Journal of Neuroinflammation* 15, no. 196 (July 4, 2018), https://link.springer.com/article/10.1186/s12974-018-1233-2; Perlmutter, *Brain Maker*, 56–57.

154. Rongzhen Zhang et al., "Circulating Endotoxin and Systemic Immune Activation in Sporadic Amyotrophic Lateral Sclerosis (sALS)," *Journal of Neuroimmunology* 206, nos. 1–2 (2009): 121–24, https://www.ncbi. nlm.nih.gov/pmc/articles/PMC2995297/; Perlmutter, *Brain Maker*, 57.

155. Judy Fulop, "High–Saturated Fat Diet Increases Endotoxemia," *Natural Medicine Journal* 10, no. 6 (June 2018), https://www. naturalmedicinejournal.com/journal/2018-07/high-saturated-fat-diet-increases-endotoxemia.

156. Perlmutter, *Brain Maker*, 49–51.

157. Maxime Fournet, Frédéric Bonté, and Alexis Desmoulière, "Glycation Damage: A Possible Hub for Major Pathophysiological Disorders and Aging," *Aging and Disease* 9, no. 5 (October 2018): 880–900, https:// www.ncbi.nlm.nih.gov/pmc/articles/PMC6147582/.

158. Fournet, Bonté, and Desmoulière, "Glycation Damage."

159. "Adult Obesity Facts," Centers for Disease Control and Prevention, June 29, 2020, https://www.cdc.gov/obesity/data/adult.html.

160. World Health Organization, *Global Health Risks: Mortality and Burden of Disease Attributable to Selected Major Risks* (Geneva: World Health Organization, 2009), v, https://www.who.int/healthinfo/global_burden_disease/GlobalHealthRisks_report_full.pdf.

161. Perlmutter, *Brain Maker*, 97, 102.

162. "The Health Effects of Overweight and Obesity," Centers for Disease Control and Prevention; "Obesity and Cancer," National Cancer Institute, January 17, 2017, https://www.cancer.gov/about-cancer/causes-prevention/risk/obesity/obesity-fact-sheet.

163. "Obesity Prevention Source: Economic Costs," Harvard T. H. Chan School of Public Health, accessed August 23, 2020, https://www. hsph.harvard.edu/obesity-prevention-source/obesity-consequences/economic/.

164. Chutkan, *The Microbiome Solution*, 61.

165. Dominique Kagele, "The 'Skinny' on Gut Microbes and Your Health," The Jackson Laboratory, May 26, 2015, https://www.jax.org/news-and-insights/jax-blog/2015/may/the-skinny-on-gut-microbes-and-your-health#.

166. Perlmutter, *Brain Maker*, 31, 98–99.

167. Kagele, "The 'Skinny' on Gut Microbes and Your Health."

168. Vanessa K. Ridaura et al., "Gut Microbiota from Twins Discordant for Obesity Modulate Metabolism in Mice," *Science* 341, no. 6150 (2013): 1241214, https://www.ncbi.nlm.nih.gov/pmc/articles/PMC3829625/.

169. "Is a Candida Infection Driving Your Sugar Cravings?," Liver Doctor, accessed August 23, 2020, https://www.liverdoctor.com/is-a-candida-infection-driving-your-sugar-cravings/.

170. "Researchers Look Beyond BMI to Predict Obesity-Related Disease Risk," Human Longevity, accessed August 23, 2020, https://www.humanlongevity.com/researchers-look-beyond-bmi-to-predict-obesity-related-disease-risk/.

171. Megan Ciara Smyth, "Intestinal Permeability and Autoimmune Diseases," *Bioscience Horizons: The International Journal of Student Research* 10 (2017), https://academic.oup.com/biohorizons/article/doi/10.1093/biohorizons/hzx015/4670557#102451706. .

172. Furness, Kunze, and Clerc, "Nutrient Tasting and Signaling Mechanisms in the Gut. II. The Intestine as a Sensory Organ."

173. Enders, *Gut*, 152–53.

174. "Autoimmune Diseases," National Institute of Allergy and Infectious Diseases.

175. "Autoimmune Diseases," Office on Women's Health, April 1, 2019, https://www.womenshealth.gov/a-z-topics/autoimmune-diseases.

176. Steven R. Gundry, "Abstract P238: Remission/Cure of Autoimmune Diseases by a Lectin Limited Diet Supplemented with Probiotics, Prebiotics, and Polyphenols," *Circulation* 37, suppl. 1 (June 29, 2018), https://www.ahajournals.org/doi/abs/10.1161/circ.137.suppl_1.p238; Gundry, *The Plant Paradox*, 38.

CHAPTER 9

1. Aimee McNew, "How Alcohol Wrecks Your Gut and 10 Signs You're Sensitive to It," PaleoHacks, accessed August 19, 2020, https://blog.paleohacks.com/how-alcohol-wrecks-gut/.

2. Enders, *Gut*, 18.

3. Enders, *Gut*, 12–14.

4. Enders, *Gut*, 119–21.

5. Enders, *Gut*, 70–71.

6. Enders, *Gut*, 119–21.

7. "Bristol Stool Chart," Continence Foundation of Australia, updated July 15, 2020, https://www.continence.org.au/pages/bristol-stool-chart.html.

8. "Water: How Much Should You Drink Every Day?," Mayo Clinic, September 6, 2017, https://www.mayoclinic.org/healthy-lifestyle/nutrition-and-healthy-eating/in-depth/water/art-20044256.

9. "How Long Is Too Long on the Potty?," Geisinger, accessed August 24, 2020, https://www.geisinger.org/health-and-wellness/wellness-articles/2017/10/27/15/44/poop-or-get-off-the-potty.

10. Dana E. King, Arch G. Mainous III, and Carol A. Lambourne, "Trends in Dietary Fiber Intake in the United States, 1999–2008," *Journal of the Academy of Nutrition and Dietetics* 112, no. 5 (May 2012): 642–48, https://pubmed.ncbi.nlm.nih.gov/22709768/.

11. U.S. Department of Health and Human Services and U.S. Department of Agriculture, "Appendix 7: Nutritional Goals for Age-Sex Groups Based on Dietary Reference Intakes and *Dietary Guidelines* Recommendations," *2015–2020 Dietary Guidelines*, 8th ed., December 2015, 97, https://health.gov/sites/default/files/2019-09/2015-2020_Dietary_Guidelines.pdf.

12. American Osteopathic Association, "Low Magnesium Levels Make Vitamin D Ineffective," ScienceDaily, February 26, 2018, https://www.sciencedaily.com/releases/2018/02/180226122548.htm.

13. U.S. Department of Health and Human Services and U.S. Department of Agriculture, "Appendix 7: Nutritional Goals for Age-Sex Groups Based on Dietary Reference Intakes and *Dietary Guidelines* Recommendations," 98.

14. M. A. Puertollano et al., "[Olive Oil, Immune System and Infection]," *Nutricion hospitalaria* 25, no. 1 (January–February 2010): 1–8, https://pubmed.ncbi.nlm.nih.gov/20204249/.

15. Gundry MD Team, "15 Steps to Reduce Lectins in Your Diet."

CHAPTER 10

1. Jennifer Hyland, "Fast Fiber Facts: What It Is and How to Get Enough," *U.S. News and World Report*, August 22, 2018, https://health.usnews.com/health-care/for-better/articles/2018-08-22/fast-fiber-facts-what-it-is-and-how-to-get-enough.

2. Brian Krans and Kristeen Cherney, "The Health Benefits of Psyllium," Healthline, April 22, 2019, https://www.healthline.com/health/psyllium-health-benefits; Alisa Hrustic, "5 Signs You're Not Eating Enough Fiber,"

Men's Health, October 30, 2017, https://www.menshealth.com/nutrition/a19540392/signs-of-low-fiber-diet/.

3. Raman, Sirounis, and Shrubsole, *The Complete Prebiotic & Probiotic Health Guide*, 63–64; Krans and Cherney, "The Health Benefits of Psyllium."

4. Taylor Norris, "What's the Difference Between Soluble and Insoluble Fiber?," Healthline, August 22, 2017, https://www.healthline.com/health/soluble-vs-insoluble-fiber.

5. Norris, "What's the Difference Between Soluble and Insoluble Fiber?"

6. "Weight Loss," Mayo Clinic, February 15, 2020, https://www.mayoclinic.org/healthy-lifestyle/weight-loss/in-depth/weight-loss/art-20044318.

7. Nicola Shubrook, "Can Constipation Weaken Your Immune System?," Constipation Experts, 2013, http://www.constipationexperts.co.uk/blog/2013/09/can-constipation-weaken-your-immune-system.html; Yu Gu et al., "The Potential Role of Gut Mycobiome in Irritable Bowel Syndrome," *Frontiers in Microbiology* 10 (August 21, 2019): 1894, https://www.ncbi.nlm.nih.gov/pmc/articles/PMC6712173/.

8. Lacy, *Making Sense of IBS*, 199–204.

9. Megan Mouw, "The Different Ways That Prebiotics and Fiber Affect the Gut Microbiota," Gut Microbiota for Health, June 19, 2019, https://www.gutmicrobiotaforhealth.com/the-different-ways-that-prebiotics-and-fiber-affect-the-gut-microbiota/.

10. Franziska Spritzler, "What to Know About Inulin, A Healthful Prebiotic," Medical News Today, April 27, 2020, https://www.medicalnewstoday.com/articles/318593.

11. Joint FAO/WHO Working Group, *Guidelines for the Evaluation of Probiotics in Food* (London, ON: Food and Agriculture Organization and World Health Organization, 2002), 8, https://www.who.int/foodsafety/fs_management/en/probiotic_guidelines.pdf.

12. Hrefna Palsdottir, "11 Probiotic Foods That Are Super Healthy," Healthline, August 28, 2018, https://www.healthline.com/nutrition/11-super-healthy-probiotic-foods.

13. Perlmutter, *Brain Maker*, 207–11.

14. "Probiotics 101: The Basics of Probiotics," Nature's Way, accessed August 25, 2020, https://www.fortifyprobiotics.com/education/probiotics-101-1.

15. Ruscio, *Healthy Gut, Healthy You*, chap. 14, Kindle.

16. Ryan Andrews, "All About Probiotics: How to Get Them from Food and Supplements," Precision Nutrition, accessed August 25, 2020, https://www.precisionnutrition.com/all-about-probiotics.

17. Mary Jane Brown, "8 Health Benefits of Probiotics," Healthline, August 23, 2016, https://www.healthline.com/nutrition/8-health-benefits-of-probiotics.

18. Brown, "8 Health Benefits of Probiotics."

19. Brown, "8 Health Benefits of Probiotics."

20. Jing Wang and Haifeng Ji, "Influence of Probiotics on Dietary Protein Digestion and Utilization in the Gastrointestinal Tract," *Current Protein and Peptide Science* 20, no. 2 (2019): 125–31, https://pubmed.ncbi.nlm.nih.gov/29769003/.

21. Andrews, "All About Probiotics."

22. R. K. Rao and G. Samak, "Protection and Restitution of Gut Barrier by Probiotics: Nutritional and Clinical Implications," *Current Nutrition and Food Science* 9, no. 2 (2013): 99–107, https://www.ncbi.nlm.nih.gov/pmc/articles/PMC3864899/.

23. Rao and Samak, "Protection and Restitution of Gut Barrier by Probiotics."

24. Kellman, *The Microbiome Breakthrough*, 112.

25. Chutkan, *The Microbiome Solution*, 170.

26. Raman, Sirounis, and Shrubsole, *The Complete Prebiotic & Probiotic Health Guide*, 41-42.

27. Ulrich Sonnenborn, "*Escherichia coli* Strain Nissle 1917—from Bench to Bedside and Back: History of a Special *Escherichia coli* Strain with Probiotic Properties," *FEMS Microbiology Letters* 363, no. 19 (October 2016): fnw212, https://academic.oup.com/femsle/article/363/19/fnw212/2236266.

28. Crystal Raypole, "Can Probiotics Help with Depression?," Healthline, March 21, 2019, https://www.healthline.com/health/probiotics-depression.

29. Raypole, "Can Probiotics Help with Depression?"

30. Reza Ranuh et al., "Effect of the Probiotic *Lactobacillus plantarum* IS-10506 on BDNF and 5HT Stimulation: Role of Intestinal Microbiota on the Gut-Brain Axis," *Iranian Journal of Microbiology* 11, no. 2 (2019): 145–50, https://www.ncbi.nlm.nih.gov/pmc/articles/PMC6635314/.

31. Brown, "8 Health Benefits of Probiotics."

32. C. Han et al., "The Role of Probiotics in Lipopolysaccharide-Induced Autophagy in Intestinal Epithelial Cells," *Cellular Physiology and Biochemistry* 38, no. 6 (June 2016), https://www.karger.com/Article/Fulltext/445597.

33. Gundry, *The Plant Paradox*, 144.

34. "How Many Times Should You Chew Your Food? (and 11 Tips for Good Digestion)," Organixx, accessed August 25, 2020, https://organixx.com/how-many-times-should-you-chew-your-food/.

35. Chutkan, *The Microbiome Solution*, 94–95.

36. Amel Taibi and Elena M Comelli, "Practical Approaches to Probiotics Use," *Applied Physiology, Nutrition, and Metabolism* 39, no. 8 (2014): 980–86, https://pubmed.ncbi.nlm.nih.gov/24797031/.

37. "Prebiotics vs. Probiotics," Jackson GI Medical, updated March 15, 2018, https://www.prebiotin.com/prebiotin-academy/what-are-prebiotics/prebiotics-vs-probiotics/.

38. Arlene Semeco, "The 19 Best Prebiotic Foods You Should Eat," Healthline, June 8, 2016, https://www.healthline.com/nutrition/19-best-prebiotic-foods.

39. John Brisson, "Arabinogalactan Prebiotic Fiber: I'm Cautiously Optimistic, a Review," Fix Your Gut, April 22, 2016, https://www.fixyourgut.com/arabinogalactan-lesser-known-prebiotic-may-help-digestive-health/.

40. "Prebiotics vs. Probiotics," Jackson GI Medical.

41. Perlmutter, *Brain Maker*, 194.

42. Adriana Rivera-Piza and Sung-Joon Lee, "Effects of Dietary Fibers and Prebiotics in Adiposity Regulation via Modulation of Gut Microbiota," *Applied Biological Chemistry* 63, no. 2 (2020), https://link.springer.com/article/10.1186/s13765-019-0482-9.

43. "Prebiotics, Probiotics, and Your Health," Mayo Clinic, May 21, 2019, https://www.mayoclinic.org/prebiotics-probiotics-and-your-health/art-20390058.

44. Leigh Stewart, "What Is Butyrate and Why Should You Care?," *Atlas* (blog), accessed August 25, 2020, https://atlasbiomed.com/blog/what-is-butyrate/.

45. Stewart, "What Is Butyrate and Why Should You Care?"

46. "Top 10 Benefits of Prebiotics and the Best Prebiotic Foods for Health," Rowdy Bars, March 4, 2018, https://rowdybars.com/blogs/rowdy-blog/top-10-benefits-prebiotics; Mark W. Hess et al., "Dietary Inulin Fibers

Prevent Proton-Pump Inhibitor (PPI)-Induced Hypocalcemia in Mice," *PloS one* 10, no. 9 (September 23, 2015): e0138881, https://www.ncbi.nlm. nih.gov/pmc/articles/PMC4580428/.

47. Xiuzhen Han, Tao Shen, and Hongxiang Lou, "Dietary Polyphenols and Their Biological Significance," *International Journal of Molecular Sciences* 8, no. 9 (September 2007): 950–88, https://www.ncbi.nlm.nih. gov/pmc/articles/PMC3871896/.

48. Megan Ware, "Why Are Polyphenols Good for You?," Medical News Today, October 18, 2017, https://www.medicalnewstoday.com/ articles/319728.

49. "The Ins and Outs of Polyphenols Supplements," Strong Health, July 6, 2018, https://www.stronghealth.com/polyphenols-supplements/.

50. "The Ins and Outs of Polyphenols Supplements," Strong Health.

51. Amit Kumar Singh et al., "Beneficial Effects of Dietary Polyphenols on Gut Microbiota and Strategies to Improve Delivery Efficiency," *Nutrients* 11, no. 9 (September 13, 2019): 2216, https://www.ncbi.nlm.nih.gov/pmc/ articles/PMC6770155/.

52. Han, Shen, and Lou, "Dietary Polyphenols and Their Biological Significance."

53. Mohsen Meydani and Syeda T. Hasan, "Dietary Polyphenols and Obesity," *Nutrients* 2, no. 7 (2010): 737–51, https://www.ncbi.nlm.nih. gov/pmc/articles/PMC3257683/.

54. Chwan-Li Shen et al., "Green Tea and Bone Metabolism," *Nutrition Research* 29, no. 7 (2009): 437–56, https://www.ncbi.nlm.nih.gov/pmc/ articles/PMC2754215/.

55. Han, Shen, and Lou, "Dietary Polyphenols and Their Biological Significance."

56. Rosario Jiménez et al., "Polyphenols Restore Endothelial Function in DOCA-Salt Hypertension: Role of Endothelin-1 and NADPH Oxidase," *Free Radical Biology and Medicine* 43, no. 3 (2007): 462–73, https:// pubmed.ncbi.nlm.nih.gov/17602962/.

57. Fernando Gomez-Pinilla and Trang T. J. Nguyen, "Natural Mood Foods: The Actions of Polyphenols Against Psychiatric and Cognitive Disorders," *Nutritional Neuroscience* 15, no. 3 (2012): 127–33, https:// www.ncbi.nlm.nih.gov/pmc/articles/PMC3355196/.

58. Gomez-Pinilla and Nguyen, "Natural Mood Foods."

59. Han, Shen, and Lou, "Dietary Polyphenols and Their Biological Significance."

60. Han, Shen, and Lou, "Dietary Polyphenols and Their Biological Significance."

61. Han, Shen, and Lou, "Dietary Polyphenols and Their Biological Significance."

62. Han, Shen, and Lou, "Dietary Polyphenols and Their Biological Significance."

63. Susan Westfall and Giulio Maria Pasinetti, "The Gut Microbiota Links Dietary Polyphenols with Management of Psychiatric Mood Disorders," *Frontiers in Neuroscience* 13 (November 5, 2019): 1196, https://www.frontiersin.org/articles/10.3389/fnins.2019.01196/full.

64. Singh et al., "Beneficial Effects of Dietary Polyphenols on Gut Microbiota and Strategies to Improve Delivery Efficiency."

65. Seray Kabaran, "Olive Oil: Antioxidant Compounds and Their Potential Effects over Health," in *Functional Foods*, ed. Vasiliki Lagouri (n.p.: IntechOpen, 2019), https://www.intechopen.com/books/functional-foods/olive-oil-antioxidant-compounds-and-their-potential-effects-over-health.

66. Kris Gunnars, "Resistant Starch 101—Everything You Need to Know," Healthline, July 3, 2018, https://www.healthline.com/nutrition/resistant-starch-101.

APPENDIX B

1. Cerner Multum, "*Lactobacillus acidophilus*," Drugs.com, June 1, 2020, https://www.drugs.com/mtm/lactobacillus-acidophilus.html.

2. Svetlana Sokovic Bajic et al., "GABA-Producing Natural Dairy Isolate From Artisanal Zlatar Cheese Attenuates Gut Inflammation and Strengthens Gut Epithelial Barrier *in Vitro*," *Frontiers in Microbiology* 10 (March 18, 2019): 527, https://www.ncbi.nlm.nih.gov/pmc/articles/PMC6431637/.

3. Erika Isolauri, "Probiotics for Infectious Diarrhoea," *Gut* 52, no. 3 (2003): 436–37, https://www.ncbi.nlm.nih.gov/pmc/articles/PMC1773578/.

4. Deguchi et al., "Effect of Pretreatment with *Lactobacillus gasseri* OLL2716 on First-Line *Helicobacter pylori* Eradication Therapy."

5. Marlene Wullt et al., "*Lactobacillus plantarum* 299v Enhances the Concentrations of Fecal Short-Chain Fatty Acids in Patients with Recurrent *Clostridium difficile*–Associated Diarrhea," *Digestive Diseases and Sciences* 52, no. 9 (2007): 2082–86, https://pubmed.ncbi.nlm.nih.gov/17420953/; Cathy Wong, "The Benefits and Uses of *Lactobacillus*

plantarum," Verywell Health, June 13, 2020, https://www.verywellhealth.com/lactobacillus-plantarum-benefits-uses-side-effects-4152035.

6. Isolauri, "Probiotics for Infectious Diarrhoea."

7. Francesco Savino et al., "Antagonistic Effect of *Lactobacillus* Strains Against Gas-Producing Coliforms Isolated from Colicky Infants," *BMC Microbiology* 11 (June 30, 2011): 157, https://www.ncbi.nlm.nih.gov/pmc/articles/PMC3224137/.

8. Evan Jerkunica, "What Is Probiotic *S. thermophilus*?," Probiotics.org, accessed August 26, 2020, https://probiotics.org/s-thermophilus/.

9. Lorena Ruiz et al., "Bifidobacteria and Their Molecular Communication with the Immune System," *Frontiers in Microbiology* 8 (December 4, 2017): 2345, https://www.ncbi.nlm.nih.gov/pmc/articles/PMC5722804/.

10. Kelli Hansen, "How to Use the Probiotic *Bifidobacterium infantis*," Healthline, May 17, 2017, https://www.healthline.com/health/bifidobacterium-infantis.

11. Toshitaka Odamaki et al., "Effect of the Oral Intake of Yogurt Containing *Bifidobacterium longum* BB536 on the Cell Numbers of Enterotoxigenic *Bacteroides fragilis* in Microbiota," *Anaerobe* 18, no. 1 (2012): 14–18, https://pubmed.ncbi.nlm.nih.gov/22138361/; Katie Stone, "Major Health Benefits of *Bifidobacterium longum*," Balance One, October 18, 2017, https://balanceone.com/blogs/news/bifidobacterium-longum.

12. Evan Jerkunica, "B. Lactics Probiotics Supplementation Benefits," Probiotics.org, accessed August 26, 2020, https://probiotics.org/bifidobacterium-lactis/.

13. Cerner Multum, *Saccharomyces boulardii lyo*," Drugs.com, November 26, 2019, https://www.drugs.com/mtm/saccharomyces-boulardii-lyo.html.

APPENDIX C

1. Brianna Elliott, "54 Foods You Can Eat on a Gluten-Free Diet," Healthline, December 29, 2019, https://www.healthline.com/nutrition/gluten-free-foods#1.

2. Katherine Marengo, "Is Soy Sauce Gluten-Free?," Healthline, December 23, 2019, https://www.healthline.com/nutrition/is-soy-sauce-gluten-free.

3. Peter Osborne, "Top Foods to Avoid on a Gluten Free Diet," Gluten Free Society, accessed August 26, 2020, https://www.glutenfreesociety.org/wp-content/uploads/Consuming-Alcohol-on-a-Gluten-Free-Diet.pdf.

4. "Is Barley Gluten-Free?," Beyond Celiac, accessed August 26, 2020, https://www.beyondceliac.org/gluten-free-diet/is-it-gluten-free/barley/.

5. Jessica Bruso, "Is There Gluten in Teriyaki?," *SF Gate*, December 7, 2018, https://healthyeating.sfgate.com/there-gluten-teriyaki-9963.html.

INDEX

DR. COLBERT'S HEALTHY GUT ZONE

prediabetes 18

probiotics 17, 23, 44–45, 55, 78, 80, 83, 100, 105, 111, 115, 120, 123, 125–129, 137, 143–144, 148, 150–151, 153, 159–166, 168, 170, 172, 175, 180, 196–197, 201, 202

Proteobacteria 6

psoriasis viii, 9–10, 12, 55, 69, 137, 141

psyllium husk 62, 80–81, 103, 109, 112, 153, 156–158, 178–179, 183, 185–186, 188–189, 191–192, 196, 201

R

Raynaud's disease 60

rectum 4, 146, 149

resistant starches 62, 145, 151, 172–173, 175–176, 180, 196

rheumatoid arthritis 12, 18, 20, 60, 68, 93, 137

rhodiola 83

Ruscio, Dr. Michael 161

S

sarcopenia 35, 94. *See also* muscle wasting

saturated fats 57, 75–78, 86–87, 131, 143, 152, 175, 177–178, 181

serotonin ix, 37, 106, 124–126, 132

shortness of breath 52–53

SIBO 12, 35, 45, 90, 95, 102, 105–112, 148, 150, 157–158, 161, 168, 180

SIFO 12, 45, 90, 101–102, 105–112, 134, 148, 157–158, 168, 180

sinus infection 9, 163

Sjögren's syndrome 60, 137

skin rashes 19

skin tags 19

small intestinal bacterial overgrowth. *See* SIBO

small intestinal fungal overgrowth. *See* SIFO

small intestine 3–4, 10, 22, 34–35, 58, 93, 95, 97, 100, 105–106, 108–110, 113, 120, 165, 167

sorbitol sensitivity 103

sphincter 92, 94–95, 97, 100, 146

Squatty Potty 81, 148

stomach vii, 4, 10, 22, 24, 33–34, 91–95, 97–101, 106, 167–168

stomachache ix, 50, 91

stomach acid vii, 22, 24, 33–35, 66, 91–96, 98–100, 106, 108, 168, 202

stress 16, 23, 57, 76, 79, 81–83, 86, 94, 97–99, 101, 117, 127, 149, 171, 173

T

tap water 39

thyroiditis 12, 55, 60, 68, 136

tight throat 52. *See also* hoarse throat

tongue swelling 52–53

Tourette's syndrome 11

transglutaminase 60

type 1 diabetes 7, 18, 60, 93, 114, 136

type 2 diabetes 77, 85, 89, 131

U

ulcerative colitis 12, 60, 90, 113, 115–121, 123, 137, 150, 168, 180, 202

ulcers 12, 23, 32–34, 89–90, 97–100, 114, 122

urinary tract infection. *See* UTI

UTI 31, 86, 163

V

vasculitis 60, 137

vital gluten 60

vitiligo 12, 19, 60, 137

vomit 52, 65, 71, 91, 98

W

water filtration system 39

weak pulse 52

weed killer 36

weight gain vii, 19, 21, 30, 35, 59, 65, 71, 95, 133–134, 154, 164, 167. *See also* obesity

weight loss x, 19, 97–98, 113–114, 116, 120–121, 135, 161, 164–165, 167, 168, 181

World Health Organization 132

242

Y

Z

MY FREE GIFTS TO YOU

I hope *Dr. Colbert's Healthy Gut Zone* helped you understand that making the right food choices will become the medicine in which you will now live and walk in divine health.

As My Way of Saying Thank You...

I am offering you two of my e-books for FREE!

- *Pandemic Protection*—E-book
- *Dr. Colbert's Fasting Zone*—E-book

To get this **FREE GIFT**, please go to:
www.drcolbertbooks.com/freegifts

Stay Healthy, and God Bless You,

Dr. Don Colbert

SILOAM